ESSENTIAL NATURAL HEALTH GUIDE
HEALTH GUIDE

FOR TRAVEL AND HOME

RICHARD PITT

IMPORTANT NOTICE

Medicine, like every other science, is subject to continuous development. Research and clinical experience broaden our knowledge, particularly as far as treatment and medical therapy are concerned. Whenever there are dosages or applications mentioned in this manual, the reader may rest assured that the author, editor and publishers have taken great care to ensure that the information given represents the standard of knowledge at the time of completion of this book.

The information in this book reflects the experience and study of the author and the information on all the remedies mentioned is widely available in standard homeopathic medical texts and other natural medicine books. However, the accuracy and effectiveness of any of the recommendations made in the book cannot be guaranteed and this book is not intended to replace professional medical care in situations where that is required. The book is designed to be used as a guide in aiding self-treatment and not as the only source of information about the given subject matter. Therefore, the authors, editors and publishers cannot make any promise of the effectiveness of any of the treatments mentioned. Readers are suggested to also consult other material and references on the subject and to consult a medical professional if indicated.

The recommended dosages and any possible contraindications are general recommendations and therefore are used at the reader's own risk. However, the authors and publishers appeal to each user to pass on any pertinent information of any reaction that comes to his or her notice.

The author and publisher cannot accept any liability for any loss or damage caused by the content of this book and make no warranties about the effectiveness of any suggested treatment. However, it is hoped that the information is of practical use to all who read the book.

Protected trade names (trademarks) are not marked in any special way. Therefore, it should not be assumed from the lack of such a mark that the trade name is free.

All rights to this manual including all or any of its parts are reserved. Any use of this manual or parts thereof outside the narrow confines of the copyright law without prior permission of the publishers is prohibited and will be prosecuted. This applies in particular to photocopies, translations, microfilms and storage and processing in electronic systems.

Title	Essential Natural Health Guide	Edition	1st Edition

www.thenaturalmedicineguide.com

Editor — Jenni Tree

Author — Richard Pitt

Printer — Edward Brothers Malloy

Design — 13² Studio, Napa, California

©2015 Richard Pitt.
All rights reserved.

Publisher — Lalibela Publishing, San Francisco, California

ISBN/EAN 978-0-976091-82-0

ESSENTIAL NATURAL HEALTH GUIDE

FOR TRAVEL AND HOME

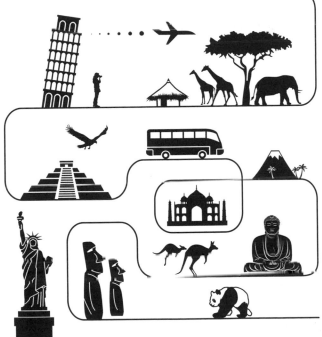

RICHARD PITT

Acknowledgements

To the many friends, colleagues and family who have supported me in this project and to all the fellow travelers, vagabonds and restless souls I have met on the way and shared special times. Thanks to one and all.

Contents

Foreword

If, like Richard you enjoy traveling roads less traveled and visiting places where you can have a real taste of a country, its people and their culture, then having a companion to guard your health and well being is more than welcome. This Natural Health Guide is the kind of companion that can follow you everywhere you go and – if not traveling – should be easily accessible on a kitchen shelf or in a bathroom cupboard.

Richard is passionate about traveling as well as natural medicine. Together with his aptitude for writing this makes him the perfect author for this book. Besides drawing from direct experience based on years of traveling the globe and decades of treating patients with homeopathy, being an avid reader he has also integrated tips from a wealth of sources making this book a rather complete guide for travel, covering a wide range of topics. As a traveler or simply being a tourist in foreign places, you can encounter many situations concerning your health. You name it and you'll find it discussed in this book.

The layout of the book is such that you can easily find the information you need for a specific situation. As making a diagnosis is not something you can always easily do yourself, the book offers you the possibility to nevertheless find a remedy to help by focusing on your main symptoms and looking for remedies there. Then by reading the suggested remedies in the back of the book you can decide what the best choice is for you based on your symptoms.

Even if you're traveling without any need to consult this book – which, being quite a traveler myself, I truly wish for you – then this book is still a great companion. While waiting on a crowded airport or at a dusty bus stop you can have an interesting introduction to natural medicine and the philosophy behind it. It also offers knowledge of how you may be able to help fellow travelers you meet while on the road, even if you are fine yourself. Isn't it great to find out that you brought this guide all the way to help him or her?

If you are not traveling much, it offers you comprehensive knowledge on how to treat many commonly seen conditions in daily life. Do grant yourself, your family members and travel companions, and those you meet on the road this practical and useful guide.

I wish you happy and healthy travels or if staying at home, a healthy life.

Harry van der Zee MD

Preface

I began to travel seriously after leaving school at age eighteen, spending four years 'on the road' between the UK and Australia, most of the time in Asia and especially India. At that time, India was a challenging place to travel in and it was very common to catch some potentially nasty stomach bugs leading to diarrhea, dysentery and worse. Hepatitis A was very common and if unlucky, malaria, typhoid and dengue fever were not unusual. Luckily I survived fairly intact, two bouts of intense diarrhea being the worst symptoms I experienced. I did get a mild dose of hepatitis A, turning yellow with jaundice when arriving home, but I soon recovered and since then all my travels have been fairly incident free. More recently I have spent nearly two years in Africa, both in West Africa and also in Malawi and Kenya. Africa has some of the nastiest diseases for the traveler to avoid, malaria being by far the most common and one of the worst. Unfortunately I did catch malaria – one bad night in a fishing village on Lake Malawi with a dysfunctional net – but I have recovered well. My experiences in traveling have made me aware of many of the challenges one can face when traveling and also simply living in your home town! This book comes out of this experience.

I did not even know about homeopathy when I was first traveling but soon after returning from my first four years of traveling at age twenty two, I began to study homeopathy seriously. I was inspired by its philosophy and through my travels and studying of world cultures, the principles of homeopathy and natural medicine made a lot of sense to me. In recognizing the healing power of nature and understanding the concept of the interconnectedness between mind and body and one's environment, the foundations of homeopathic theory connected with me and I thought that if these ideas and principles can be applied directly in the practice of medicine, they must have huge potential. Thirty years later, my experience has confirmed this initial inspiration. I have seen amazing results, both in chronic long term diseases in my practice and also working in the field in Africa and India. I have seen people who are writhing in pain in front of me get better in a matter of minutes when the right remedy is given. This is not an uncommon experience. It has given me the confidence to be able to recommend homeopathy and natural medicine for a wide variety of conditions that anybody can come across.

I have been practicing homeopathy now for over thirty years, initially in England and then in the United States. Although most of this work has been treating chronic conditions found in western cultures, I have also treated many infectious, acute conditions. From over eight years of travel in most parts of the world, I have had the opportunity to use homeopathy in many acute conditions not often seen in the west. I have worked with local communities and have helped establish schools and teaching programs for people to learn the fundamentals of homeopathic practice. I have also studied homeopathy and spent time with homeopathic practitioners in Greece, India, Australia, New Zealand, Brazil, Africa, Europe and North America. This book is a result of my own experience of practicing homeopathy and of traveling extensively over many years. Most of the natural health options discussed in the book are therefore homeopathic remedies, which can be bought in convenient kits for travel and for storage at home, as well as some important herbal medicine options to complement the homeopathic suggestions. Hopefully this information will give confidence to travel far and wide, knowing that many possible health issues can be addressed effectively.

The information in this book can add to your arsenal of health options, both away from home and also for basic day-to-day health issues.

Introduction

The purpose of this book is to give clear and simple options that homeopathy and other natural medicines have to offer for a wide variety of acute conditions. These are particularly relevant at times when traveling and also for first aid use in the home. However, I felt the need also to include situations which are potentially more serious, especially when traveling in challenging areas. Given the limitations of conventional medicine and access to appropriate medical care, especially in more remote places, knowledge of how to treat many simple and some complex health issues is as important today as ever. Homeopathic medicine especially has a good track record in treating many of the conditions mentioned in this book.

The success of homeopathy was clearly documented, first in Europe in the 1820's and 1830's during cholera and typhoid epidemics, as well as in the United States during the deadly flu pandemic of 1918, where statistics showed that homeopaths had a death rate of only 1.05%, in comparison with over 30% under allopathic care, and even up to 60% at times*. In the 1st World War in the United States there was a homeopathic medical corps, staffed by 100 nurses, 22 physicians and two dentists, nearly all homeopaths. In 1922, President Harding, whose father served as a homeopathic physician in the Civil War, hosted a convention of homeopaths at the White House. In the late 1800's in the United States, there were 22 homeopathic medical schools, 100 homeopathic hospitals and over 1,000 homeopathic pharmacies.

Today, homeopathy is an integral part of the health care systems of many countries, including India, which has over 20 homeopathic medical schools, South and Central America where homeopathic departments exist in public hospitals in places like Rio de Janeiro, most of Western Europe, South Africa, Australia, New Zealand etc.

Homeopathy has solutions for numerous epidemic diseases both old and emerging, as well as for many other diseases. This book is designed to give you access to some of this valuable information. The recommendations in the book however, are not designed to take the place of conventional medical care. Homeopathy can be used along with all other forms of medical care, conventional and otherwise. In any situation, the risks need to be weighed up in deciding the best course of action to take. Ideally this book will help you to be able to evaluate these risks and to know what course of action to take.

Homeopathy is a well proven system of medicine that has been practiced all over the world for over two hundred years. There are now professionally trained homeopaths and people seeking homeopathic and other natural medical care in every continent, including Africa, most of Asia, Europe, North and

South America, Russia and China. If you would like to look at the developing body of research into homeopathy, you can find it at the Homeopathy Research Institute **www.homeoinst.org**, among other sites. A basic introduction into the philosphy and principles behind natural medicine is given on the website **www.thenaturalmedicineguide.com**. It is highly recommended to read this in order to gain a basic foundation into homeopathy and other forms of natural medicine. This can help give an understanding how to appropach using the remedies suggested for many conditions.

The first two chapters give an introduction on how to use homeopathy and natural medicine in general and an overview of how to prepare for various forms of travel and how to avoid many illnesses. As mentioned, using homeopathic and herbal medicine does not take the place of conventional care and often both methods may be used at the same time. However, having simple and effective natural methods available can greatly help when health challenges arise. Each condition needs to be looked at carefully and if any condition in the book is potentially serious, recommendations to get a professional opinion or care are given.

The therapeutic chapters begin in Chapter Three with accidents, injuries and trauma and cover most accidents and first aid situations one can experience. It also covers some specific travel experiences, including jet lag and travel sickness. It is followed by a chapter on the treatment of emotional conditions. This chapter is given priority as homeopathy can effectively treat emotional conditions and the connection between emotional and physical states is important to understand when using homeopathic remedies. Chapter Five focuses on digestive conditions, which again are some of the most commonly experienced ailments found when traveling. Ideally, many of these conditions can be avoided by taking precautions outlined in Chapter Two, but sometimes one simply can't avoid getting sick. The following chapters cover a wide range of conditions including more serious tropical diseases and infections. The book is designed to be succinct but detailed enough to cover most diseases one can come across, when traveling, and also at home.

The website **www.thenaturalmedicineguide.com** also gives an outline of all the prevention methods one can use for many conditions, including a comparison of vaccines available for various diseases and natural options that can be used instead or in conjunction with vaccines for various diseases. The risks of various forms of travel are discussed so people can evaluate the level of rsik they are taking for various forms of travel. It is important that every person traveling knows as much as possible about the types of diseases they could face and what options are available to avoid getting them. The site also has information on where you can find homeopathic remedies and other resources throughout the world.

Chapter Nine gives a list of 52 remedies mentioned in the book and their main symptom picture. (A more comprehensive list of remedies is found on the website but this list covers the main remedies found in homeopathic travel medicine kits).This chapter can be used as a reference and complements the information in each chapter. Some remedies are mentioned a lot in many chapters and for many conditions. Having knowledge of the key points for the most popular remedies can greatly help in recognizing when these remedies are needed. This obviously comes with experience, but ideally this book can help in the study of important homeopathic and herbal remedies used.

I hope this book helps you in your knowledge of how to use homeopathic and herbal medicines and gives you confidence to use them, wherever you are in the world and in whatever circumstances you are in.

*Perko, Sandra, *The Homeopathic Treatment of Influenza: Surviving Influenza Epidemics and Pandemics Past, Present, and Future with Homeopathy*, Benchmark Homeopathic Publications, San Antonio, Texas (1999).

Essential Natural Health Guide

Chapter One
How To Use Natural Medicine

How to read this book

Each chapter deals with a variety of similar conditions connected by similar causes or which are found in the same region of the body. For each condition, a number of homeopathic and herbal remedies are suggested, along with a brief description of the condition and how it occurs. A detailed list of all the remedies recommended in the book are found in Chapter Nine and should be used to complement the information given for each condition. Each remedy may be used for more than one condition and it is useful to have an understanding of the main characteristics of each remedy. The more familiar you are with the qualities of each remedy, the more easily you will recognize them in yourself and friends when they are needed.

The information presented is not meant to take the place of conventional medical care or the advice of your physician. However, it does offer an alternative to conventional care if that care is not working or is not available. Homeopathic and herbal remedies can also be used in conjunction with other alternative and conventional medicines. For each condition, a number of homeopathic remedies are suggested, followed by other natural approaches that can be used at the same time. It is not always easy to find the correct homeopathic remedy for a condition as there are often different possibilities. This book attempts to simplify that process for the reader and make the choice of remedy that much easier. If it seems difficult to choose the correct remedy, the reader has to pick one remedy or put more than one remedy together by mixing them in water and taking or giving it in a liquid form. Directions of how to give the remedy(ies) will follow.

Homeopathic remedies are not only given according to a disease diagnosis but to a unique group of symptoms, which can be potentially seen in many different disease states. It is important to recognize the key qualities in each medicine and identify those key features when they appear in a particular condition. For example, the remedy *Arsenicum album* is useful in both diarrhea and also various fevers, but one has to see some qualities of burning pains, restlessness, anxiety and chilliness to justify the remedy, whatever the condition and name of the disease. However, not all the symptoms of a remedy have to be there to give that remedy. A select few is enough but the symptoms have to be the most characteristic ones that the person is experiencing and that are found in the remedy.

All homeopathic remedies are given their Latin name. This is consistent throughout the world. Homeopathic remedies can be found in many countries, including all of Europe, the United States,

Central and South America, Canada, Australasia, India, Pakistan, Bangladesh, Sri Lanka and Russia. In most countries, the remedies will be made according to strict criteria and are trustworthy. If you are in any doubt, please consult a homeopathic consultant and ask them. Homeopathic remedies are freely available to buy in most countries, either from pharmacies or natural food stores (if they exist). Otherwise, you can purchase them through homeopathic doctors. *See website for details of how to access remedies.*

How to take homeopathic remedies

In general, you can give/take one or two globules/tablets, put it/them into your mouth and let dissolve. It doesn't matter though if you chew it. Do not take anything else at the same time as you take the remedy, including water, tea or coffee. Take the remedy dry. Ensure your mouth is clean and has nothing else in it. Only handle it if your hands are clean. Otherwise, use the lid of the bottle. Do not touch a remedy if it is for somebody else.

If a remedy is to be repeated frequently (more than twice a day), it is best to dissolve one or more globules/tablets into two to four ounces of water and take one teaspoon according to the frequency indicated, which depends on the severity of the symptoms. Even a remedy to be taken three to four times a day can be done this way and, each day, make a new batch with fresh water and another globule/tablet. The water should be stirred or shaken well each time before taking a teaspoon of the liquid. It makes no difference in terms of strength if the remedy is taken dry or in liquid form.

If a tablet is dissolved into a small amount of water, the imprint of the remedy is infused into the water and it will have the same effect as taking a tablet on the tongue. What is important is the potency/strength of the remedy and how often it is repeated.

In more extreme situations, e.g., a high fever or intense pain, a remedy can be taken every one to five minutes, or every fifteen minutes to every hour, depending on the situation. You can't really take too much of a remedy. Your body will take what it needs and when symptoms subside then you can simply stop or reduce the remedy. In more chronic situations, like an old strain or injury, then taking one tablet daily for one week will be enough. It will need some time to see major improvement. On average, you will be taking or giving a remedy one to three times a day.

The same applies to the potency (strength) of the remedy. Each homeopathic remedy is given a number after its name. This relates to the potency of the remedy and the strengths are often as follows - 6c, 30c, 200c, 1m and 10m. The higher numbers relate to a higher or stronger potency and are usually used in more serious conditions. However, for practical purposes, only 30c and 200c are recommended here as these are potencies that come with kits and that are more widely available. They are also strong enough for most situations. Some remedies have the letter X after them. See the end of this chapter for more explanation.

Some remedies may be mentioned that are not included in the kits used with this book. These remedies would have to be purchased separately, either locally or online. A list of all the remedies mentioned in the book and in the kits available are on the following website:

www.thenaturalmedicineguide.com. If you think that one of the remedies listed could be needed, due to particular travel plans or prior experience, then it is good to get this remedy in advance.

Alternatively, you may want to consider some herbal medicines to complement the homeopathic remedy given. The dosages will also depend on the severity of the condition and instructions should be followed for each condition, which are found on the label of all herbal preparations. Generally, homeopathic and herbal preparations can be given in conjunction with any conventional medicines being taken but especially with herbal preparations it is important to pay attention to any potential interactions between the two. If you have any questions, do consult your prescribing doctor and read labels of all preparations.

How to take herbal remedies

Herbal remedies should generally be taken according to instructions that come with them if they are bought in a packaged form. However, given that herbs are physical substances with possible side-effects, it is important to note any effects and to stop if symptoms are getting worse or new conditions develop. It is also important to follow any recommended information for children and pregnant women. If herbs are taken in a loose form, being made up on the spot or in places where it is not possible to evaluate the dosage, caution should be taken and it is good to start with a small amount and note the effect and gradually build up if it seems fine to do so. It is also worth asking people who have experience with local herbs.

How to keep remedies safe

Homeopathic remedies will stay effective for an indefinite amount of time if they are looked after, irrespective of any expiry date on the label, which is done to comply to law. They should be kept in a water proof container and be kept as dry as possible. Sometimes in the tropics they can get moist but try and keep them dry. Do not expose remedies to direct sunlight or very strong smells, like eucalyptus, camphor etc. Avoid too intense heat. If pills escape and fall to the table or floor, do not put them back in the bottle. Prolonged exposure to X-rays may antidote the remedies. However, it is now unavoidable if one travels by air as all baggage is X-rayed. It seems that remedies work well after exposure to X-rays when traveling, but it is worth paying attention if much travel is done over a number of years as their strength may be eroded over time.

Evaluating the action of homeopathic remedies

Homeopathic remedies will generally work according to the needs of the body. In intense situations in which there is a high fever, acute pain or some other very acute situation, the remedy will work in between one and fifteen minutes. In less severe situations, some change will be seen in one to four hours. For example, in a sprained ankle without much pain, relief will be seen in twelve hours to two days. A simple case of diarrhea may take one day to get better. A more intense case may take longer but some improvement in most cases will be seen in the first day. One does have to have some patience though. Do not panic just because you have diarrhea and take every over-the-counter medicine possible. Give the body a chance. One has to assess the needs of the situation to the action of the remedy.

In intense situations, when a remedy works, the first reaction is often that the person falls asleep. This is a good sign. Once there is a clear sign of the remedy working, then the remedy can be stopped or given less frequently. Use your judgment. If pain disappears totally, stop the remedy. If symptoms begin to return, begin the remedy again, repeating at suitable intervals. There is some flexibility here. If a remedy is working, do not change it. Continue it less frequently until it has completed its action. Also, consider a higher potency of the same remedy if it initially worked well and then seems to stop working.

Sometimes the remedy is only partially effective as it is not the exact one needed, but it will still work somewhat and perhaps another remedy will follow to finish things off. Pay attention to how well a remedy works and always keep other possible remedies in mind. Look at the other remedies listed for the same condition.

One of the first signs of improvement is an increase in energy and well being, even if the symptoms persist. This is good. In time the symptoms will get better. If symptoms seem to get a little worse immediately after taking a remedy, it is usually a sign that the body is being activated through the remedy and relief should soon set in. The rule generally is that the more intense the situation, the quicker the remedy will work. It may take only seconds to see relief or it may take a number of hours and even days in situations that are more long term.

Trust the remedy. If it is correct it will work and it will work quickly if need be.

Terminology

- **SD** Single dose (usually taken once daily).
- **Allopathy** Term used in homeopathy to describe conventional medicine.
- **Acute condition** A self limiting condition that may often require support but will normally resolve by itself in time.
- **Chronic condition** A longer standing condition that normally will not resolve by itself, requiring homeopathic constitutional care by a professional, or some other form of therapy.
- **Constitution** Relates to the basic physical and psychological characteristics of a person.
- **Nosode** A homeopathic remedy made from diseased material, e.g., discharge from bacterial infections.
- **6x, 12x, 6c, 30c and 200c, 1m, 10m** This relates to the strength of the homeopathic medicine. Potencies with an X (or D) after have been mixed in a ratio of 1/10 (that is one drop of the substance mixed with 10 drops of water). Those with a C after have been mixed in the ration of 1/100. Take each remedy as indicated but if a 200c is indicated and you only have a 30c or 30x or even D12, then take that instead. In this book, only c potencies are being recommended, mostly 30c and at times 200c, but if you can only get x potencies somewhere, that will work fine.

Chapter Two
Being Prepared

It is useful to research the types of health challenges one can face in the countries being visited. This way, you can be forewarned and take all necessary precautions. This is not just for medical reasons but also to understand the culture you may be visiting and the various norms of that culture, including food habits.

Many of the conditions found in this book are only found in certain areas of the world. Knowing the likelihood of getting any of these diseases can help you in your preparation and to know what preventative measures to take. Also, if you have particular nutritional needs, knowing what foods may be available may also be important. Eating local food is often one of the interesting parts of travel, but is also one of the riskiest activities in terms of getting sick.

If you are embarking on more arduous journeys requiring special preparation, then doing the necessary research ahead of time is invaluable.

Avoiding getting sick is the best strategy when traveling or for that matter, at any time. Most diseases travelers get are passed on through contaminated food and water. By far the most common conditions experienced are some form of diarrhea due to bad food, more so than water. Therefore being prudent in this area is crucial for well being.

Other forms of prevention can involve taking natural medicines, supplements and also conventional medicines. One of the most common forms of conventional prevention used is vaccinations or immunizations. Discussion of vaccinations with their risks and benefits and natural options are given on the website *www.thenaturalmedicineguide.com*.

Minimize infections

It is impossible to avoid coming across a multitude of infectious agents when traveling, especially in more challenging places. Part of this is due to our contact with unfamiliar bugs we have little immunity to and partly the circumstances we find ourselves in, especially eating out and the hygiene challenges we may come across. However, the body is generally quite resilient and after a while, some natural immunity is developed. But it is not uncommon when traveling to get at least one dose of diarrhea or a cold of some sort.

However, take all precautions to prevent infection. Wash your hands a lot, especially before and after eating. Take your own liquid soap with you. Also you can use anti-bacterial wipes or gels to prevent infections although I have never done so myself. This is useful though when water is not available or if you have to use water and your hand to clean yourself after going to the bathroom. This is a very common practice in much of the world and is very hygienic as long as you can wash your hands afterwards. Don't walk barefoot apart from on beaches. You can catch various little creatures and also injure your feet, which is often a source of infection in tropical areas.

Food and Water

It is imperative to avoid drinking bad water or contaminated food. They account for a majority of diseases travelers get on the road, including diarrhea, dysentery, cholera, typhoid, hepatitis A etc. Bad food is sometimes harder to avoid now than bad water, so particular attention should be given to the food eaten. Drink bottled water or boil your water. Also take water sterilization methods with you. Iodine or chlorine is best. Even cleaning your teeth in tap water should be avoided unless you know the water is OK. In restaurants plates and cutlery can still be wet and should be wiped clean. Carry a clean small towel or wipes with you.

Common sense is important. Always check out the places to eat and where you get your water from. Research the good bottled water companies. They are not all the same. Also, sometimes there are scams to refill empty water bottles so check the lid is sealed and the water tastes OK. Some water tastes like gasoline due to the process of filtering and sterilizing. Do not drink it. Luckily, this happens less now than it used to. Do not put your lips to any bottle that somebody else has drunk from. Avoid ice and ice cream as this is very risky. Commercial soft drinks are generally OK and sodas can be useful to help a mild upset stomach. Some local brands may not be that good and can at times have nasty chemicals in so it is best to ask around what people drink. However, it is best not to drink too many sodas and to hydrate with water and other natural liquids. Fresh coconut water is excellent for hydration and general health.

Badly prepared food is the major form of catching bacteria, viruses and parasites. It is important to check out as much as possible the quality of a place before eating. The following are a few hints.

- Eat where locals eat, (within the boundaries of normal hygiene). Does the place seem busy and active.
- A fancy restaurant does not necessarily indicate a clean kitchen but avoid 'dumps'.
- Avoid any food that tastes 'bad'. (I know that sounds obvious but at times we continue to eat something we shouldn't. Meat and fish particularly need close attention).
- Avoid uncooked food, including salads (unless you can be sure it has been cleaned thoroughly). Especially avoid lettuce. Peel all raw vegetables and fruit. Avoid mayonnaise as it may carry salmonella. Fresh yoghurt is OK but even then, be careful.
- Avoid raw or undercooked meat or fish in any form. It is best to stick to a more vegetarian diet in many countries. Meat is often not kept in a hygienic way and is a vector for some very unpleasant bugs. Fish can also be a problem, especially shell fish. If eating fish, ensure it is cooked well

Essential Natural Health Guide

and generally avoid shell fish. Avoid all fish caught in contaminated waters, for example, during red tides (when many fish die for various reasons and pollute the sea). Always check with locals what fish are good to eat. All milk should be boiled before drinking. Even boiled milk left to cool can quickly become infected. Minimize consumption of dairy food and eggs.

- Avoid food that has been re-cooked or re-heated, including rice. Fried rice is very suspect as often it is slightly reheated from a previous meal. If food is meant to be hot, make sure it is hot when you eat it.
- Eat what the locals are eating. Do not ask for foods that they are not that familiar with.
- Don't pick your own berries or other wild food – including mushrooms - unless you are sure you know what it is. It may look like a plant back home but it could be poisonous.

Discussions and theories about basic nutrition are seemingly more complex than religion. Endless theories about diet are continually being debated with 'new' diets constantly emerging, whether for weight loss or optimal nutrition. Modern agricultural methods are producing vegetables with less of the essential vitamins and minerals we need and it is debatable if many people, even in developed economies, are getting enough essential nutrition. Therefore a good quality vitamin and mineral supplement, (which are food based as opposed to synthetically based) is recommended as part of one's daily nutrition. However, when traveling it is not crucial to take supplements with you especially if traveling for only short periods. There is fresh food easily available in most developing countries and the diet may be simple but fairly healthy.

If you eat meat, then ideally you should know where it comes from and what the animal is being fed. That means eating locally produced organic meat. The industrial meat industry, especially in the United States, is producing meat full of hormones and antibiotics. They are often kept in horrendous conditions, which must affect the quality of meat, let alone the ethical considerations, making eating such meat a health risk. Eating organic meat is much more important than eating organic fruit and vegetables. However, especially in the United States, the introduction of genetically modified (GM) foods into the food supply makes eating organic and local produce more important. In spite of all the ideas floating around about diets and the importance of nutrition, it is fair to say that if one sticks to eating as many vegetables as possible and a reasonable amount of fruit (in tropical climes, fruit becomes a greater proportion in ones diet), eating whole grains mainly (brown rice, quinoa, oats), pulses (lentils, all sorts of beans) and small amounts of fish and meat if you choose to, is a good diet. Avoid too much dairy and use olive oil for most cooking. Coconut and sesame oil are also good. Avoid all margarines and also canola oil which are too processed. Palm oil is fairly ubiquitous in Africa and parts of South America, but this should be used sparingly and has environmental problems in its production. Ghee (clarified butter) is common in India and is generally fine. Avoid too much sugar, although this is easier said than done in many countries.

However, at home, it is not so hard. Wean yourself off sugar in your coffee and tea if you can. There is a growing epidemic of diabetes in both developed and developing countries. Diet is a major factor.

Hydration

It is very important when visiting warm humid countries to stay hydrated. Drinking enough is crucial for well-being and to avoid dehydration. This is especially the case when exerting oneself and sweating a lot. So make sure you drink enough water. Take your own water bottle with you, ideally made from stainless steel. Plastic bottles deteriorate and the hard plastic bottles leach chemicals over time and when exposed to the sun. If you do become dehydrated, for whatever reason, drink small amounts to begin with. Do not drink too much at first. However, before any exertion, walking in the heat etc., take in as much water as you can. Prevention again is the best option. Once you have drunk a lot before exertion, resist taking in more water until you really have to. If you do drink more water, most of it is simply sweated away. Drink only when you really need to if you are dealing with a limited water supply. Pay attention to the symptoms of dehydration - dark, odorous urine, difficult respiration, stiffness of joints, excessive tiredness. Carry rehydration tablets with you if think there is any chance of becoming dehydrated.

Rehydration can help with many conditions. Obviously treating a disease like cholera requires instant rehydration, but even for situations like jetlag, altitude sickness and tiredness from being in a hot, tropical situation can benefit from using rehydration mixtures. Any diarrhea that continues more than 24 hours or is particularly intense is a good reason to use them. However, with any diarrhea, simply drink more water and other fluids. Do not drink milk. If you don't have rehydration mixtures, use the following equation: one teaspoon of salt with eight teaspoons of sugar and one liter of clean water. You don't want it too salty. If making a smaller amount, use a pinch of salt to one to three tsp. of sugar. Honey, brown sugar, molasses etc., are fine to use instead of white sugar. You can also add a pinch of salt to a soft drink instead. It may taste bad, but it will work. Generally avoid hot drinks to rehydrate, but lukewarm drinks are OK, including various teas and even weak coffee. Do not drink alcohol to attempt to rehydrate.

If you feel dizzy or have a headache with diarrhea you may be dehydrated and you have to drink more. Oral rehydration mixtures (ORS) can be taken if you are a diabetic but an acute diarrhea may upset sugar levels.

Adjusting to a very warm climate can be one of the most challenging things for those unused to such climates. The heat can be enervating and some constitutions are very challenged by such situations. This is why it is crucial to maintain your water intake. Drink a lot.

Ensure the water is clean. If offered a glass of water that has not been treated, refuse unless you are sure it is OK. Take a cup of tea instead. Even if that water is not totally boiled, hot water still kills many bugs. Boil your water before drinking. Boil for about two minutes. If at higher altitudes, boil the water longer. For example at

5,000 ft, boil it for at least five minutes. Once the water is boiled, do not put it into an untreated or used plastic bottle. Do sterilize any water bottles you are using by pouring boiling water into them.

If it is not possible to boil the water and no other treated water is available, get a plastic bottle, put some water in it, and leave it in the sun for about five hours. In that time, many of the bugs would be killed. If the water is still murky one can filter it through a sock if the material is woven tight enough. This is just in emergencies. There are various forms of filtration equipment that are effective in cleaning water of most bugs. However, they are often awkward to use and carry and are not always that effective. They are more useful as part of using chemical sterilization or when you will be in one place for quite a while, instead of moving around a lot. However, some portable filter bags are useful to have if you are in the 'bush' and the water is particularly murky. Chemical sterilization is useful to have if you are doing any kind of traveling in areas where you cannot find access to good bottled water. It is worth finding out ahead of time what the situation is in the places you may be going to. The two main forms of sterilization are using chlorine and iodine. Both work. Chlorine tastes worse. They may not kill cysts that can cause dysentery and giardia unless the dose is high enough (five to ten drops per liter or one tablet per liter). However, do check this information when buying chlorine or iodine equipment.

If you are sweating a lot, you should ensure that you are getting enough salt. Simply use more salt on your food. Normally your body will crave more salt but pay attention to this and use a little more. A refreshing drink to take is carbonated or still water, with fresh limes or lemons squeezed in and a pinch of salt.

Travel

The actual process of travel takes its toll, from stiffness and sleeplessness to travel sickness and the need to be aware of deep vein thrombosis (DVT). Any long trip should involve being able to stand, stretch and loosen up the body. Especially stretch the legs by pointing the feet forward and then flexing the feet back. A DVT comes when due to blood collecting in the lower limbs, a clot forms which then travels up the body into various organs, which can kill. So, especially when traveling by air, make sure you get up frequently, stretch and walk about. Also to avoid DVT, stay well hydrated and avoid wearing tight socks. Jet lag is another common experience, which cannot really be avoided but can be minimized by staying hydrated, minimizing alcohol and by trying to sleep. Taking a natural or conventional sleeping aid may be useful in helping to get some sleep. *See Chapter Three: Jet lag section* for remedy choices for both prevention and treatment.

If you are feeling sick when traveling or know you get travel sickness or have been sick and then have to travel, take precautions before your journey. Consider taking conventional medications to prevent nausea and sickness. Take some plastic bags with you just in case! *See Chapter Three: Accidents, Injuries and Trauma, Travel Sickness section.*

Heat

One of the big adjustments to tropical travel is dealing with the heat, especially humid heat. Many parts of the world, including Latin and South America, Africa and Asia have very hot climates and for those from northern climes, it can be overwhelming. Some people deal with heat much better than others. Overexposure to the sun and heat in general should be avoided. Dehydration, as discussed, is a major risk of travel and you need to be aware of this at all times especially when exerting yourself in hot climates. Give yourself some time to adjust to a new climate on arrival. Don't rush out on the first day and overdo it. There can be a tendency to want to have air conditioning wherever you stay, but it is best to resist this. Going from one extreme to another is not healthy and you do not adjust to the heat so easily. There are times when it can be a refuge, especially if the nights are extremely hot but do not overdo the A/C option. Wearing a hat can be invaluable when out in the sun and if you dampen it, it can help you stay cool. Make sure you take one with you. Balding heads are particularly susceptible to sunburn and it doesn't take long to get burnt.

Equipment and supplies

Being prepared before travel saves a lot of time. If you are traveling and suddenly need something, it often becomes a hassle to find it. This is both for basic supplies as well as medical equipment. While this book is focusing on natural medicine for both travel and home, having a good basic medical kit with you is very helpful.

Also, ensure you take the right clothing. Shoes especially should be worn in before leaving, particularly if trekking. Take a good pair of sandals and/or flip flops, which are useful to wear in showers and other 'dubious' places. However, don't feel you have to spend a fortune on all sorts of travel gear, even if trekking. There can be a compulsion to be over prepared and you end up carrying way too much stuff. Often you can figure out what you need when you arrive, unless you really know certain things are not going to be available there.

In terms of general supplies you should always include the following: (This is mainly a list that also pertains to health. There are many other individual items you may need and have to be prepared to have).

- 2 torches (flashlights), one hand held and the other attached to the head. You should take AA or AAA batteries or take a wind up flashlight which doesn't use batteries.
- Enough batteries to fit your devices. They are not always easy to find or of good quality when traveling.
- Alarm clock or cellular phone. Ensure the phone is unlocked so you can get a local SIM card if traveling for any length of time.
- Pens - enough for yourself and to give away. Ball point pens make excellent gifts for children.
- Electronic reader - Ipad, Kindle, Nook etc. Given the ever increasing restrictions on weight allowance when flying, this can be especially useful and also, as long as you have access to a wireless connection you can get downloads. It is also good for guidebooks if you don't want to lug one with you as

well as medical information and this book.

- Stainless steel water container (minimum of 1 liter).
- Map of the area traveling in. Often they are better quality in your own country than where you are visiting.
- A small travel towel that dries quickly. I always travel with an Indian wrap around 'sarong', which serves as a towel and also for general wear whenever you need to put something on.
- A wash cloth. Very useful when having a bucket wash and using a limited amount of water.
- A pocket knife (with scissors). Tweezers if not part of the knife.
- Sunscreen if you will need it but only use it when necessary. People tend to lavish it on their bodies because of fear of skin cancer. However, unless you are at high risk or have moles that may turn cancerous, it is best to use sunscreen only until you have turned brown and then decrease its use. Most sunscreens are fairly toxic. There is also some evidence that using sun glasses all the time may lessen your skin's ability to adapt to the sun, so the skin gets more easily burnt. This is due to the lack of melanin being released to the skin as the sunglasses give the impression to the brain that you are not in the sun. Fairer people and those whose skin is more at risk should always be careful in the sun.
- Sunglasses, if you are going to be in very bright sunlight for prolonged periods of time. Increased cataracts are a direct result of too much light exposure, e.g., hiking in high altitudes and in the snow. However, as mentioned,

they do not need to be used for general sunlight unless you are particularly sensitive to sunlight. Ensure you get good quality glasses.

- Spare reading glasses.

Medical supplies

- Insect repellent: A DEET based repellent (30-50%) is important in malaria infested areas. Clothes, especially socks, can also be soaked in repellant for extra protection. A roll-on stick or spray is most efficient. I find the sprays more messy. Natural insect repellants such as citronella and eucalyptus mixed together in an alcohol based spray can be used as a daily repellent and should be taken as well and is nicer on the skin than DEET which I try to use only on clothing. Other natural sprays can also be used.
- Mosquito coils (although these are commonly found in most mosquito infested places).
- Antiseptic wipes.
- Band-aids of various sizes and some non stick dressings and tape. Steristrips. Blister aids if walking a lot (moleskin, and special tape for blisters).
- Oral rehydration (ORS) if you are going to be in remote and/or very hot places.
- Hypodermic syringes, just in case you need injections and you don't want to be using old syringes.

You may choose to take some conventional medications with you in case of emergency. This can include antibiotics to treat local skin infections, respiratory conditions and the variety of digestive issues commonly experienced. It may also include antihistamines and some painkillers. You should consult your doctor before traveling as to what is possible and appropriate. If going to tropical areas, it may be better to consult a tropical specialist. However, ideally most conditions can be treated with natural medicines and antibiotics etc., can be saved for emergencies only. Don't feel the need to take strong antibiotics at the beginning of any condition. Also, be careful buying medications abroad. In developing countries, many can be fake or dangerous, so only buy from a reputable source.

Chapter Three
Accidents, Injuries, Trauma

It is important to pay attention to any injury and treat it accordingly. Homeopathic remedies have an affinity for various types of injuries, whether a blow or a cut and also for certain types of tissues e.g., ligaments and muscles, and areas of the body. It is useful to know which remedies address the different tissues of the body and the nature of injuries they cover. It is always important to pay close attention to any injury in case of shock or damage to internal parts of the body and bleeding. What may seem superficial may in fact be a more serious injury. More than one remedy may be needed to affect a cure. Always treat the physical and or mental shock first before going to other remedies. Most likely this will be *Arnica* in physical shock and *Aconite* in mental shock. Please look at the various subsections below for more information.

Accidents and Injury

This is a catch all phrase to cover the variety of situations which need to be treated due to a trauma to the body, including injuries to bones, ligaments, tendons and muscles. It is amazing how effective homeopathic remedies can be in treating all forms of trauma, including sporting injuries and also just the physical stress from over exertion. Prevention is better than cure and taking necessary precautions before strenuous exercise is important. Try not to overdo things at the beginning of any physical exertion. Be prepared, drink and eat enough and don't put your body through too much stress. It can take days to recover and limit your enjoyment and ability to enjoy your experience. Take homeopathic *Arnica* to help prevent stiffness and exhaustion from too much exertion. If you know you are going to over-exert yourself, e.g., competing in a long run or cycle ride, take *Arnica*, one tablet a day for up to three days before the event and three times a day during the event.

If you get wet through from walking through rivers, lakes or due to any other factors, have another set of clothes to change into. Don't stay too long in wet clothes. Be prepared. If you get really chilled, get warm as soon as possible. If you get seriously chilled and can't get warm, take homeopathic *Aconite* (see below).

Even when an injury is more serious and muscles, tendons, ligaments or bones are damaged, homeopathic remedies can facilitate their healing and speed recovery. Different types of injuries are given their own subsection below, but as you will see, many of the same remedies are indicated for different injuries. It is worth reading the whole section to get a good idea of the images for each remedy and the types of injuries covered.

● HOMEOPATHIC CARE

Arnica is the first remedy at the beginning of any injury. It is the best remedy for any physical shock or blow, especially with bruising, including injuries to the breast. If you are trekking, it is useful to take it during the first day of hiking when it is easy to overdo it. Take one tablet two to three times that day. Often people walk much further than they should and suffer the consequences. *Arnica* will help here. If you feel any soreness and bruised feeling with any injury, especially to soft tissues, take *Arnica* first. *Bellis perennis* is needed in breast injuries if swelling and nodules remain. *Arnica* is also the first remedy for any concussion. Often you can think things are OK and you may say everything is fine when it is not. If you are around any injury in which a person says they are fine, give *Arnica* and wait and observe. If, after an injury there is more emotional shock, with residual fright.

Aconite is the first remedy to give if there is more emotional shock and fright, or fear remains after a trauma or accident. One tablet hourly for four hours should be given before considering other remedies for the physical injury

Ledum is needed if bruising and swelling does not go away after a few days or only is partly helped, especially in cases of a black eye with residual swelling or bruised feeling, or in injuries to soft tissue, joints and muscles. It is the first remedy to give for punctured wounds and swelling, whether a bite from an insect or a penetrating wound like a nail. It helps prevent tetanus. It is also good for sprains to joints, with puffy swelling and a cold feeling of the injured part.

Hypericum is needed in penetrating punctured wounds, when pains are extreme and shooting from the injured part, It is excellent for injuries to nerve rich areas where the pains are shooting, sharp and very intense, e.g., injuries to fingers and lacerations to nerve rich areas as well as injuries to the spine, especially the coccyx and the back of the head (occipital).

Rhus tox and *Ruta grav* are remedies to consider when the injury is more to the muscles, ligaments, tendons and joints. If you have any kind of joint or muscle sprain, whether a hamstring, or injury to the elbow, shoulder, ankle or knee, then these two remedies are important. There can often be a sore, bruised, stiffness in the injured part, which is better through moving it for a while, but then becomes worse from overuse. There can be swelling in the injured area but often the pain improves with warmth. *Ruta grav* is the first remedy for tennis elbow and simple eyestrain from too much reading and is indicated in injuries to smaller joints, like wrists and ankles. *Rhus tox* is indicated for larger joints and muscles, e.g., shoulder joints and hamstrings.

Bryonia is useful for injuries involving joints and bones and often is used in alternation with *Rhus tox.* In *Bryonia*, initially you do not want to move the injured part at all. Everything is made worse from any motion and you want to keep it totally still. Later, as stiffness becomes stronger, then movement may make it feel better, indicating *Rhus tox. Bryonia* can be given when there is a broken bone when any movement is unbearable.

Symphytum is excellent for broken bones. Commonly known as knit bone, it helps unite bones once they have been set. It is good for fractures of the cheek bone.

Calendula is a remedy applied locally in a tincture and/or cream as well as an internal remedy. It is useful for any wounds, especially cuts, lacerations and punctured wounds. It is a great healing agent and antiseptic. Some tincture should be put into warm water and the injured area cleaned thoroughly. Internally it is given in a tablet form when lacerations are very painful.

NOTE More than one remedy can be needed and often it begins with *Arnica* and then moves to another remedy, depending on the nature of the symptoms and the exact tissues most affected.

🖉 HERBAL CARE

Calendula cream and comfrey cream are used for open wounds. If wounds are deep though, a tincture of calendula should be used instead. Lavender, eucalyptus and tea tree oils also can be used.

Altitude Sickness

Symptoms include dizziness, nausea, fatigue, confusion, weakness, headache, breathlessness and palpitations. Symptoms may be acute and quite sudden or gradually develop. This can be a life threatening condition and should not be neglected.

● GENERAL CARE

Do not ascend more than 2,000 feet (600 meters) in one day where you intend to stay overnight. If symptoms are intense, then slowly descend to a lower level of altitude. Do not overexert yourself. Drink a lot of water. You have to avoid any dehydration.

● HOMEOPATHIC CARE

Coca is the first remedy to consider. Take one tablet every thirty minutes until relief. If that doesn't work or you don't have that remedy, take *Arnica* every thirty minutes. (As *Coca* is made from the plant that cocaine is derived from, it is not so easily available over the counter in pharmacies, even though the homeopathic dosage is just a highly diluted form of the plant).

● HERBAL CARE

Chewing coca leaves may have the same effect as the homeopathic *Coca*. (Please check for legality in regards to taking coca leaves. For example, taking coca leaves in Peru may be fine, but it is not OK to take them across the border to Brazil). Taking coca tea works best.

Bites and Stings

The treatment of bites partly depends on what has bitten you. Most nasty bites are from creatures that emit poisons, the most serious being jelly fish, spiders and snakes. However, various insect bites can also be quite serious. Secondary infection of bites, especially in tropical areas is an important consideration and care needs to be taken. Most bites are not serious however. The localized area often becomes swollen and can be painful. This is the natural reaction of the body. In itself, it is not a cause for concern, although any bite needs to be appropriately cleaned to prevent infection. One particular type of bite needs to be discussed is a dog bite, especially in countries where rabies exists. If there is any doubt, you must see a physician and have it checked out. One other important factor is the possible diseases that the bites can spread. This is especially the case for diseases such as malaria, yellow fever, dengue fever, Lyme disease, etc. Lyme disease comes from a bite from a tick and is prevalent in the Eastern regions of the United States, parts of Europe and increasingly other areas. Woodlands and grassy areas where deer are found are the most frequent places of infection.

See homeopathic care for treatment suggestions and Lyme Disease in Chapter Six.

● **GENERAL CARE**

Ensure any bite or sting is clean. Initially the bite (or wound) should be cleaned well with warm water and soap, washing the wound for at least five minutes. In the case of a bite from a dog the wound should then be washed in alcohol (isopropyl alcohol or even vodka) to further clean the wound, *Calendula* tincture and/or *Echinacea* tincture should also be used. If any insect bite is stinging and burning, use *Urtica urens* tincture or cream or any other natural relief for stings. You can also use tea tree or lavender. There are bites from flies that can be very painful and need both local and internal treatment. Also some flies called botflies or tumbu flies can lay larvae that burrow under the skin and can be very painful. If you come back from tropical parts and seem to have something that looks like a cyst under the skin, get it checked out. If still in the tropics try and bring the larvae to the surface by putting paraffin on the infected part or again try using essential oils like tea tree. For leeches, try and remove them by either scraping them off the skin, putting tea tree oil on them or salt. Once removed, use some tea tree or calendula solution to clean the wound. If you are walking barefoot in water and stand on a sea urchin, put the skin of a papaya on the wound and it will help extract the spine of the fish. Otherwise, getting it out can be difficult and painful.

● HOMEOPATHIC CARE

Apis and *Ledum* are the first remedies to consider for the effects of simple bites. *Ledum* is the main remedy for punctured wounds of all sorts, including that of animal bites, including ticks. The local area may get puffy and swollen, which although may be red in color, may even feel cold. It is best to start with this remedy if no other remedy stands out. *Apis* can either follow *Ledum* or be given first if the bitten area is red, swollen and hard, and has stinging or burning pain. *Apis* will often be needed for the stings of poisonous animals, such as wasps and bees and also if there is any kind of systemic allergic reaction to any bites. In case of a systemic reaction to a bee sting, medical intervention may be necessary. The worst case scenario is a person who goes into anaphylactic shock. This needs immediate medical intervention but *Apis* can be given every one minute while getting attention. In the case of tick bites, once the tick is removed, give one tablet of *Ledum* 30c, twice daily for one week. You can also give one dose daily for one week of the remedy *Borrelia*, a nosode made from the Lyme bacteria.

Hypericum can often follow *Ledum*, especially when the bite or sting is very painful and pains shoot along the nerve endings from the area of the bite. *Lachesis* can be needed when the bite looks as though it is becoming infected, turning a bluish/purple or black color or becoming abscessed. You may feel intense burning or stitching pain in the wound. This is often due to venomous bites, especially of snakes and spiders.

Belladonna should be given if there is any bite from a dog, merely as a precaution against rabies. Also, *Lyssin* (a nosode made from rabies) should also be given if possible, both remedies together, one tablet two times daily for one week. However, conventional anti-rabies injections should be taken if there is any risk of the animal having rabies.

Snakebites
including spiders, scorpions, jelly fish etc.

The effect of snake bites depends partly on the type of snake doing the biting and also the amount of venom that infects the body. The local skin reaction to a snake bite does not necessarily indicate its toxicity. Also, it is not always clear from the wound site if poisoning has actually taken place. Classically the bite marks of a snake are two fang holes, about 1.5 cm or more apart. However, even one fang hole can indicate poisoning. Any wound similar to this needs to be checked and precautions taken (see below). The main physiological action of snake venoms is a hemotoxic (blood) and neurotoxic (nerves) effect. Overall, most bites from very venomous snakes have a death rate of around 20% if left untreated. The time of the bite till death varies between five hours to two days. At times, with smaller snakes, the wound may not be that obvious and can initially be ignored. However, the smaller snakes may have some of the most virulent poison. It is imperative to get medical help as soon as possible as a precaution. Also take necessary precautions if in an area where poisonous snakes are found. Wear appropriate clothing and shoes, make noise when walking and pay attention. Know the behavior of snakes in the area being visited and find out where and when the greatest risks are.

Most spider bites are not that dangerous and can be treated as any other bites. Occasionally more serious symptoms can develop with occasional fatalities. The most common and quite serious spider bite is from the black widow (Latrodectus mactans), the female of which inflicts the serious bite. They are found in most parts of the world where the weather is warmer. They can often be found under toilet seats in outdoor lavatories and can therefore bite the genitalia. Although the bite itself is hardly felt, within minutes there can be acute symptoms of intense pain in many parts of the body, with spasms through the whole body within an hour. It may seem as if the person is having a heart attack. There may be great difficulty breathing. Symptoms are mostly better within two days. A more severe bite comes from the Sydney funnel web spider (Atrax robustus) which can aggressively pursue its victim and is found in urban areas of Australia. Immediate medical attention is needed with these bites. One spider that creates a necrotic effect of its bite is the brown recluse spider (Loxosceles reclusa). The bite becomes an ulcer, the affected part being 'eaten away' by the venom, leaving much scarring. It can take months to heal. Each of these spiders are homeopathic remedies in their own right but will not be the first line of remedies used. The remedy *Tarentula cubensis* (Cuban spider) can be considered for the ulcerative effects of the funnel web spider as can *Crotalus horridus* and *Lachesis*, both remedies made from snake venom.

Scorpion stings can be very painful and create much local pain and swelling in some cases, but are not as lethal as other bites. However, some scorpions have a more neurotoxic affect and therefore it can have more serious consequences, with symptoms of pain, difficult respiration, sweating and even convulsions.

Jelly fish stings are quite common and are mostly not serious. However, the most serious sting/bite of any creature is from the box jellyfish, found predominantly off the coast of Queensland in the north east of Australia during the summer months, December to July. It is imperative to avoid being stung by these jellyfish. More common is the sting of the Portuguese man-o-war, found in many parts of the world. The sting is intense, with pain and burning of the part. More systemic symptoms can arise, including nausea, vomiting, headache, and a general feeling of shock.

See Shock section and Chapter Seven: Skin Conditions, Ulcers section.

● **GENERAL CARE**

Clean the wound well, with water, soap and an antiseptic, (***Calendula*** tincture, alcohol etc.). Follow with ***Echinacea*** tincture to the wound. If the bite is on the arm or leg, tightly bandage the whole limb and keep it still. Do not move unduly. Do not attempt to suck out the poison. If the bite is on another part of the body, clean and apply a bandage, maintaining some pressure on the part if possible. Get medical attention. If a snake bite, the offending snake should be killed so that the appropriate antivenin can be given. The antivenin is made from the venom of the offending snake species. A general antivenin may be given if the identity of the snake is not known. In jelly fish stings, putting vinegar on the sting helps as can urinating on the sting. Also, meat tenderizer can be used on the sting, especially if you prefer that to urine! However, urine may be more immediately accessible!

◆ **HOMEOPATHIC CARE**

Aconite is the first remedy to give when there is a great emotional shock and fright from the bite. Once the shock has subsided, you can follow on with other remedies.

Essential Natural Health Guide

Lachesis is the most likely second remedy to give, as described above. *Crotalus horridus* (a remedy made from the venom of a rattlesnake) can also be considered when the local swelling becomes blue/black and the blood from the wound is also black. The snake remedies are considered more when there are serious toxic effects of poisonous bites. *Echinacea* (in tincture or homeopathic potency) can also be given along with or instead of *Lachesis* for the toxic effects of bites, especially when the affected area looks infected and gangrenous.

Apis is needed when the area is puffy or hard, red, hot and stinging and *Ledum* if the part feels puffy but cold.

Arsenicum album is needed when there is much burning of the affected part and you feel very chilly and restless and also perhaps feel very anxious and fearful about the situation. In these situations, the remedy needs to be repeated very frequently, between every five to thirty minutes, depending on the severity of symptoms.

COMBINATION STRATEGY If the symptoms are more physical and local, with swelling and red discoloration of the part, begin with *Apis* and also *Ledum*. If it quickly becomes dark blue/purple, give *Lachesis*. If it develops more into looking gangrenous, add *Echinacea*. If burning is predominant, give *Arsenicum album*. If necessary, mix all together in water and take every ten to fifteen minutes for two to three hours. If anxiety and shock are predominant, begin with *Aconite*. Repeat the remedy in water every five minutes for up to one hour. Add *Arsenicum album* if *Aconite* is not enough to relieve the anxiety.

🍃 HERBAL CARE

For snake and spider bites, mix clay powder with water to make a clay pack and add a little goldenseal powder or lavender oil. *Echinacea* tincture should be taken internally.

Burns

Burns need to be treated seriously and with great care. It is important to know the degree of severity of the burn, whether it is a first, second or third degree burn. Second and third degree burns often need urgent medical care, especially if a larger area of the body is affected. Any burn which is larger than the size of a hand should have professional medical care. All burns need to be kept clean and free from infection.

● GENERAL CARE

Simple first and second degree burns, affecting a small, local area.

Remove any clothing or material that is burning the skin but leave any material that has already been totally burnt. Also leave any dead skin on the burn. Do not peel off. Do not pierce any blisters on second degree burns. Use cool or even slightly warm water to cool the area down. Do not use cold water. (The application of slightly warm water or warm heat may seem contradictory but if done in small frequent applications, it will relieve the burning pain. This is applying the homeopathic law of similars, Like cures Like). If the burn is a second degree, try and soak the burnt part in cool water. Apply homeopathic burn cream or any burn cream once it is dry but not too much to make it too moist. If possible keep the burnt area as still as possible. Ideally do not cover the burn unless there is a risk of infection due to the need to move, travel etc. If so, then place appropriate gauze bandage (non adhesive) loosely to the burnt area and keep in place with a loose bandage. Do not tie too tightly, obstructing the air getting to the burn, which will help it dry and heal. Use the cream frequently to aid the healing process. Also Vitamin E or Aloe vera gel can be used, in conjunction with the burn cream as needed. For sunburn, you can put avocado on the skin to help soothe it. Also coconut oil can be used on the skin, both as a slight sunscreen and also to soothe the skin after the sun. You can also rub coconut meat onto the skin after being in the sun. The sap from an unripe papaya can be used if the burn looks infected, 5 drops of sap and one tablespoon of salt in one liter of boiled water, left to cool.

Second degree burn of a larger area or third degree burn.

Seek medical advice and also use homeopathic remedies as described below. Do not interfere with the burn in any way. Use cool water on the burn area and keep the person still. If possible, soak the burn for 15 minutes. Using a spray bottle, spray diluted *Calendula* tincture over the burn. Do not use creams initially. Cover the burn with appropriate sterile padding if available or use cling-film or a plastic bag. Do not wrap around but put on in layers. Do not let the sterile padding or any clothing become dry on the burn area. The plastic helps avoid this and you can wrap moist cloth in plastic if that is what you have. Keep moist (with clean water) until medical attention is found or if in more remote situations and there is no help, then keep a moist padding on the burn area while the pain is intense. Eventually you will have to let the area dry and treat as above for first degree burns. Use damp clothing (but not wet) if no padding is available but again keep it moist to avoid sticking to the burn area. Chemical and electrical burns need medical attetnion.

● HOMEOPATHIC CARE

First degree and simple Second degree burns.

Arnica can initially be given for at least two hours (one time every thirty minutes) to address the shock of the burn. *Arsenicum album*, *Cantharis* or *Urtica urens* can be given to address the burn.

Cantharis is the first remedy to consider when one feels intense, burning, scalding pains, and where blisters are forming on the burn. Onc can feel in an agitated, frenzied state.

Arsenicum album is needed when there is great anxiety and restlessness with the burning pain. *Urtica urens* is useful in simple first degree burns with little other symptoms.

Second degree (larger area) and Third degree burns.

Aconite is needed immediately after a more serious burn, to address the mental shock. The remedy should be given every five to ten minutes while medical attention is being sought.

Cantharis should then be given once the shock has subsided and repeated every thirty minutes for six to eight hours and then less frequently until the pain is under some control. This may take a while.

Causticum should be given, once daily for a week if there are any chronic affects of a more serious burn, especially with feelings of great rawness still in the burnt area. *Radium bromatum* can be considered for burns due to X-rays and other radiation exposure.

🌿 HERBAL CARE

Use some honey with a little lavender oil. Spread liberally over the burn area. Rescue remedy (a *Bach* flower remedy) can also be taken for the shock. Aloe vera gel is excellent to help relieve sunburn.

Sunburn

Try to avoid getting sunburn. When initially in the sun, pace yourself. Only stay in the sun for short periods at a time. Be aware that you often don't know you are burnt until it is too late. Areas where there is little fat on the body get burnt more quickly. Use good quality sunscreen until you are brown. If you are have pale skin and/or many moles on your body, pay close attention and do not let yourself get burnt. If you notice a mole changing shape, becoming irregular, getting bigger or changing color, get it checked by a doctor.

If you are burnt, get out of the sun. Cool off under a shower but do not use cold water. Use cool water to the burnt part. Once dry, use homeopathic burn cream and/or after sun lotion. Keep cool and hydrated. If more serious, then treat as for normal burns.

Concussion

Concussion is due to a blow to the head, resulting in some level of confusion and/or temporary unconsciousness. What may seem like a light blow can in fact be concussion. It is important to check to see if there is a possibility for concussion and get medical advice if in doubt. Many people who strike their head say they are fine when they are not.

● GENERAL CARE

If no medical advice is immediately available then sit the person down. Assess if they are confused or not. Look into their eyes. Check to see if one pupil is larger than the other (there may be fluid in the cranial cavity), whether they can follow your finger with their eyes and if they can stand OK. Give them time to recover. Check for headaches, nausea or vomiting, change of pulse or respiration, mental dullness or confusion.

◆ HOMEOPATHIC CARE

Arnica is the first remedy to give for any concussion. Give one tablet every 30 minutes for at least three hours and wait.

Cocculus. is needed if there is still some dizziness, confusion and heaviness in the body and the head feels too heavy to hold up, give If that doesn't work and there is much trembling of the body and heaviness of the eyelids, give *Gelsemium*.

Natrum sulphuricum is indicated for chronic complications of a head injury, even years ago, especially if it is chronic headaches or mental depression and anxiety. you can give one tablet a day for three days.

Emergencies and Disasters

There are times when some situations become very extreme and out of control and in such intense times, using homeopathic and other natural remedies may literally be a lifesaver. Even when living in fairly safe places, one never knows when something extreme can occur, for example, natural disasters such as tsunamis, floods, fires, earthquakes, volcanoes etc. Or, if witness and exposed to other forms of emergency disasters, e.g., car, boat or plane accidents, extreme violence in war situations, or exposed to toxic chemicals or air pollution e.g., radiation, fire fumes, oil, chemicals in water or the air etc. There are many situations that are out of our control which if we are in the wrong place at the wrong time can profoundly affect us. Knowing which remedies that can be used can be crucial in these times.

◆ HOMEOPATHIC CARE

Aconite and *Arnica* are indicated for the initial stage of any trauma, *Aconite* is for acute mental shock. *(See Shock section and Chapter Four: Emotional Conditions). Arnica* is for physical shock. *(See Accident and Injuries, Concussion, Fractures etc.)* Both these remedies can be given very frequently, (one tablet dissolved into a glass of water and one sip taken every one to ten minutes) as necessary in acute situations. The more intense the situation, the more frequently the remedy can be taken.

Aconite may often be used with *Stramonium* in a situation where extreme violence is being observed or if one has been threatened by violence and tremendous fear and terror remain. *(See Chapter Four: Emotional Conditions, Fright section.)* The remedies in the Shock section are also good to know and can also be thought of in any emotional trauma.

Aconite and *Gelsemium* are needed in the event of experiencing and surviving a natural disaster like an earthquake. If there is a state of collapse or unconsciousness, both from shock or from some physical trauma, *Arnica* is the first remedy but also *Arsenicum album*, *Camphor* and *Carbo veg* are important remedies. *See Fainting and Shock sections.*

Arsenicum album is one of the first remedies to consider if there has been overexposure to some form of toxic chemical, e.g., radiation, chemicals, chemotherapy or other poisons, *(See Poisoning section)*, especially if there are any burning pains, along with acute restlessness and fear. It is excellent for burns to the skin, or burning of the mouth, esophagus and stomach from ingesting chemicals and for intense nausea from radiation or other chemical poisoning.

Ipecac is also excellent when chemicals have been ingested, as it helps to purge the body to get rid of the toxicity. *Nux vomica* is also strongly indicated in cases of poisoning when there is much retching, vomiting and spasms in the digestive area..

Radium bromatum is needed if there is great burning of the skin and of the joints after radiation poisoning. It is also a remedy for X-ray burns to the skin, along with *Phosphorus*, which also has digestive symptoms from radiation therapy. There is even a homeopathic remedy made from X-ray which can also be used for similar situations and often for chronic skin and organ problems that stem from X-ray exposure. However, constitutional care with a professional is needed in such situations.

Fainting

It is important to know why a person faints. It is due to a lack of blood supply to the brain, and can often happen due to low blood pressure or from emotional stress. It is useful to consult a doctor if it is a recurring condition as some people are more prone to it than others.

● GENERAL CARE

If you feel faint, simply sit down and put your head between your knees. Breathe slowly and deeply and wait. Often when stressed, we forget to breathe. If a person has already fainted and is unconscious, simply keep them horizontal, on their side and ensure they have loose clothing and breathing is not impeded. Do not try and rouse them.

◆ HOMEOPATHIC CARE

Aconite is the first remedy to give if fainting is due to any shock, especially sudden and intense fright. *Gelsemium* can also be used if dizziness and trembling are experienced. *Ignatia* should be used if fainting is from emotional shock, such as grief or sudden loss. *Cocculus* is used when fainting is due to lack of sleep and general exhaustion.

Ignatia and also *Coffea* are useful if fainting arises from too much excitement. If it occurs after being angry, then give *Nux vomica*.

Fractures including dislocation

Most fractures require professional care as soon as possible. Depending on the type of fracture, bones may need to be reset and appropriate structural support given. A fracture is more obvious when the bone is at an unusual angle or there is a distinct shortening of the limb. However, sometimes the break is a compaction and so will not be so obvious. However, the intensity of the pain, bruising and swelling with inability to move very much and pain on any motion may lead to the diagnosis of a fracture.

● GENERAL CARE

In any injury where any movement brings great pain, keep very still and avoid any unnecessary movement. This includes injuries to the spine if there is any chance of a break. In the case where movement is necessary, support the injured part with appropriate measures like an improvised splint or bandaging to minimize motion of the part. You should ideally refer to an appropriate first-aid source for how to do this well.

● HOMEOPATHIC CARE

Arnica, ideally in 200c potency can be given straight away, especially if there is much swelling and bruising.

Bryonia is needed when any motion brings great pain, and in this case frequent doses are needed, every fifteen minutes until some relief is felt. It is the first remedy to consider for a dislocation of a joint, along with *Arnica*. The remedies can be alternated if necessary. The remedies should be repeated very frequently as needed. If in a fracture, *Arnica* has been given and there is not much swelling but the pain.

Eupatorium perfoliatum is given if pain remains after giving *Arnica* for a fracture. one tablet, three times daily for at least three days for the pain. *Symphytum* should be given once the bone has been reset and in place. This can be given once daily for up to two weeks. It will help unite the bone.

Frostbite

Frostbite is due to freezing of parts of the body, usually the extremities and mostly when mountaineering. The frozen part should ideally be thawed slowly if possible. If more serious, then thawing should only be done if refreezing of the part is not going to happen as that can make things worse. Frostbite can also occur at warmer temperatures when the extremities become very wet and also if there is a lack of circulation.

● GENERAL CARE

Any clothing should be dried out as much as possible, including boots. If the part is numb, gentle warmth should be applied, but not excessive heat. If the feet are affected, then ideally you shouldn't be walking far. If the skin breaks, then *Calendula* or *Hypericum* tincture should be added to warm water and a bandage dampened with the warm water mixture and applied to the part.

● HOMEOPATHIC CARE

Agaricus muscarius is a specific remedy to help with frostbite, including the burning, numbness and tingling often experienced. If that does not work or is not available, then use *Lachesis* instead. Give one tablet four times daily for three to five days.

Hangover

Many people at some time of their life have drunk too much alcohol and suffered the consequences. There is often nausea and/ or vomiting and a headache. Mentally there can be great irritability and a desire to stay quiet and alone.

● HOMEOPATHIC CARE

Nux vomica is the most specific remedy for a hangover. It is one of the great remedies for the after effects of alcohol and the over-sensitivity experienced.

Headache

Headaches are caused by many factors. Headaches of a chronic nature require more constitutional treatment to understand the underlying causes. The only headaches addressed here are due to either trauma, heatstroke, poisoning, including alcohol, and acute emotional states.

● HOMEOPATHIC CARE

Belladonna, *Gelsemium* and *Glonoinum* are the main remedies to consider for headache due to acute heatstroke or any affects from the sun. *(See Heatstroke section)*. *Nux vomica* is the remedy to think of for alcohol or other poisoning, *Arnica*, *Cocculus* and *Natrum sulphuricum* if from head trauma. *(See Concussion sections)*. *Ignatia* can be thought of if due to acute emotional upset and grief.

Heatstroke
including sunstroke and heat exhaustion

Heatstroke (sunstroke) is a condition due to over exposure to sun and often combined with either a lack of fluid intake, excessive alcohol consumption or an inadequate amount of salt in food. It is potentially a very serious condition and can lead to a rapid rise in temperature, nausea, vomiting, collapse and even convulsions. This requires emergency medical intervention.

More commonly found is heat exhaustion, which is not so extreme and occurs from being in the sun too much, and also being dehydrated after exertion. Symptoms often found are dizziness, exhaustion, headache, cramping of muscles, nausea and vomiting. The temperature is much less high than in heatstroke and the person can often feel cool, with shivering. One critical difference between the two is that in heatstroke, the skin tends to be dry and it may be hot and red, whereas in heat exhaustion, it is usually cooler, paler and with more sweat.

Sun headaches are quite common, although some people are much more prone to them than others. The underlying sensitivity to sun exposure requires constitutional homeopathic care.

● GENERAL CARE

Due to the increased intensity of the sun, we all have to pay close attention to being over exposed to direct sunlight. It is important to avoid too much exposure. Wearing a hat and keeping hydrated is important. Use good quality sunscreens as necessary. The sun is not bad and some exposure is fine, but not too much all at once.

In more serious heatstroke cases the person must be put onto the ground if unconscious and bathed with cool sponges. The temperature should not be reduced too quickly. Clothing should be removed and the person ideally covered with a wet sheet and fanned. If conscious, put a damp cloth around the head, neck and extremities. The temperature should be taken frequently, every ten minutes. Once the temperature has lowered to around 103f, this treatment can be stopped. The remedy *Carbo veg* (one tablet put in water, one sip taken every minute) should be given at the same time and **Belladonna** or **Glonoinum** can be followed: see below. Medical attention is necessary.

In heat exhaustion, the person should be allowed to sit or lie down, and to be rehydrated with water and salt (for every half liter, put ½ tsp of salt and four to six tsps of sugar – or in one cup of water, put a pinch of salt and one teaspoon of sugar). Drink slowly and gradually. If you are feeling weak, dizzy, nauseous and not sweating much when in the sun, then take precautionary measures as soon as possible. Rest in the shade for quite a while and rehydrate. Be careful as further exposure to the sun, even days ahead may lead to further problems. Also, be careful with alcohol consumption when in intense heat.

◆ HOMEOPATHIC CARE

Glonoinum and **Belladonna**. are two main remedies indicated in heatstroke and acute consequences from being in the sun. In **Glonoinum**, there is the most intense throbbing, exploding headache, as if the head is going to blow up. The face is hot and flushed and the blood feels as if it is rushing to the head. It is a remedy for extreme congestion of the blood. There can be violent palpitations, which are worse from any motion or jarring. It is the first remedy to think of when there is unconsciousness due to heatstroke. **Belladonna** is the other remedy to consider for such extreme situations but also for simple sun headache when there is heat and throbbing of the head and body. The pupils can be dilated and a fever, which if very intense, can even include delirium. It is very similar to *Glonoinum*, but *Glonoinum* is even more intense, with more violent congestion.

Gelsemium is very good for sun exhaustion. In this situation, there is exhaustion, and feeling achy and dizzy and at times confused, disoriented, drowsy and chilled, often with trembling *(See Shock section)*.

Hemorrhage

Hemorrhage is any form of unnatural bleeding. It is important to know the reason why a hemorrhage is occurring and to seek professional medical care if there are any doubts. The following remedies can be considered for different kinds of hemorrhage and can even be given while on the way to getting medical care.

◆ HOMEOPATHIC CARE

Arnica is the first remedy for any hemorrhage due to injury e.g., nosebleed or from any other orifice. There can be great bruising of the skin and soreness. *Hamamelis* is another remedy for bleeding which can be used if *Arnica* doesn't work. It is great for bleeding hemorrhoids and bleeding gums after tooth extraction and nosebleeds after a blow. The flow of blood is often dark, persistent and may be oozing.

Ipecac is a remedy for any bleeding associated with nausea, especially uterine bleeding of any sort, particularly after childbirth or miscarriage. It is also used for nosebleeds with coughing and nausea. The blood is often bright red and profuse. *Phosphorus* can also be given when bleeding occurs very easily, again with bright red blood and like **Ipecac** is needed after childbirth or from uterine fibroids.

Belladonna is useful for any bleeding where the blood is bright red and hot and the face feels hot and red with a pulsating pulse.

China is good when bleeding is associated with fainting and weakness. It may be from the uterus or from the rectum with diarrhea. **Mercurius** is useful for bleeding from the rectum with diarrhea *See Chapter Five: Digestive Conditions, Dysentery section.*

⊘ HERBAL CARE

Shepherds Purse (**Thlaspi bursa pastoris**) tincture to 6x. For uterine hemorrhage, with cramps and colic, whether from a miscarriage, labor and post labor. Follow instructions on the label on how to take if in a tincture. If in a homeopathic potency, take one tablet three to five times daily for two days.

Jetlag

This is a common condition that most people experience to some extent. Some people however are much more affected by it than others and if so, it is good to take some remedies preventatively to minimize symptoms. Altering one's watch to read the time at the destination may help to relieve jetlag!

● GENERAL CARE

When flying, it is important to keep hydrated and to minimize alcohol content. Dehydration is a major factor in jetlag, especially in long haul flights. Drink a lot of liquid. Also put a little more salt on your food and/or take rehydration salts. It is important to keep moving during long haul flights to stop the possibility of deep vein thrombosis.

◆ HOMEOPATHIC CARE

Arnica can be taken three times the day before the flight for general preparation if you experience jetlag normally. *Cocculus* can also be given in this way if you feel the following symptoms from jetlag – weakness, heaviness and dizziness and even hollowness in the body, especially the head.

Cocculus is one of the great remedies for problems from a loss of sleep, and if one suffers a lot from losing sleep, then this remedy is indicated. *Nux vomica* is for when one feels hung over, and is oversensitive to noise and feeling irritable and touchy.

Carbo veg can be thought of, especially after long haul journeys and one feels simply exhausted, flat and tired and if one's digestion is bad, with gas and bloating.

NOTE You can take whichever picture most fits your experience with jetlag, even just before flying. You can also often find a combination homeopathic remedy called NoJetLag at airport shops and take that if you have no other remedies.

Pain

It is important to find out the reasons for any pain. There are good homeopathic remedies for a variety of pains and will be found discussed in the regions affected or the conditions associated with the pain. It is important to know exactly what the pain feels like and how the person, even if it is you, is dealing with the pain. Do you want to keep still, move around, shriek, weep or become angry with the pain? This makes a difference which remedy may be needed. As always, getting professional care can be important to understand what is going on.

● HOMEOPATHIC CARE

Chamomilla is one of the great remedies for pain used in homeopathy, especially in children. Pains seem unendurable, with much crying, even shrieking and anger. This is seen in abdominal colic, teething pain and fever. It is as if the reaction is well beyond what it should be.

Coffea is another pain remedy, especially teeth pain but also colic and other pains. There can be great oversensitivity, and great restlessness and weeping with the pain. *Nux vomica* is also similar to both these remedies and the pain is intense, cramping and spasmodic, and seen with anger, intolerance and great sensitivity.

Bryonia is a great pain remedy, especially for broken bones and injuries where the slightest motion creates intense sharp and bursting pain.

Hypericum is the remedy needed for nerve pains, especially injuries to nerve rich areas, e.g., fingers being trapped in doors, lacerations to nerve areas, back injuries etc. Pains are sharp, shooting, violent, feeling intolerable. *Arnica* is the remedy given when the pains always feel sore, as if bruised.

Colocynthis is excellent for acute abdominal colic, doubling the person up and needing to put great pressure into the abdomen. It is the remedy when colic comes on after suppressed anger.

Magnesium phosphoricum is very similar and a great remedy for all spasmodic pains, colic and cramping pains, all of which come on suddenly and which change place frequently. There are neuralgic pains better from heat and pressure, including toothache and colic. Pains can extort cries. The person can be constantly talking about their pains.

Poisoning

● **GENERAL CARE**

At times, accidental poisonings occur, either due to intake of toxic chemicals (something children can do inadvertently) and also by eating poisonous mushrooms and other plants. Medical intervention is ideally required, especially if the toxic dose is large or the person is becoming unconscious. It is very useful to know what type of poison has been taken. In general, the poison needs to be purged from the body and an emetic can be given to do this. Salt and warm water will work well, using at least one tablespoon of salt to a large glass of water. It should be drunk quickly to encourage frequent vomiting. If it is mushroom poisoning, then salt and water should not be given but vomiting should be induced with an emetic like *Ipecac*. Also some of the mushroom species ingested should be collected for examination later. If the poisons are corrosive chemicals, then emetics should not be used but alkaline liquids given such as Milk of Magnesia can be taken.

Other forms of poisoning include the ingestion of chemicals and also the after effects of conventional medicine, in the form of chemotherapy and radiation. Remedies can be given to help in such situations. Miso soup has been known to be effective in helping to detoxify from exposure to radiation. Japanese people have been using this method.

◆ HOMEOPATHIC CARE

Arsenicum album is needed if there is intense vomiting and purging already taking place. This can be followed by *Veratrum album* if there is cold sweat on the forehead. If the person is in a state of collapse, then *Carbo veg* should be given. *(See Shock section)*. *Aconite* can be given if there is a lot of anxiety and fear. However, professional care should be sought as soon as possible.

Arsenicum album is one of the first remedies in cases where toxic drugs have been taken, including the use of chemotherapy (and radiation) for cancer, when there is great nausea and burning pains in the body, especially in the digestive sphere. *Phosphorus* can also be considered.

Sepia and *Tabacum* are two other important remedies when extreme nausea is felt. In *Sepia* there is nausea which is much worse from the smell and taste of food but also can be better after eating food. In *Tabacum* there is intense nausea with a sinking and deathly feeling, a cold sweat and at times a collapsed state.

Shock

Shock can be either physical or mental. Both issues are dealt with here. This also includes situations when a person has collapsed. In mental shock, the person is normally conscious but often in a state that includes profound agitation, disorientation, confusion, fear with shaking, rapid heart-beat and dizziness etc. The cause of the shock can be varied, from being in or seeing an accident, or an earthquake or some other natural trauma or disaster; or from experiencing violence, both verbal and physical, or anything sudden and extremely intense. *(See Concussion, Fainting and Heatstroke sections and Chapter Four: Anxiety and Grief)*

● GENERAL CARE

Physical shock or collapse may come from simply fainting or it can be due to more serious and intense physical conditions, such as a heart attack. It may also be due to a loss of blood or the affects of physical trauma. Often the person is either semi-conscious or unconscious. In either case, the first thing to do is to take care of the person. They need to be placed in a horizontal position on one side and to ensure they can breathe freely. If the person is not breathing, then resuscitation should be given. (A first aid course should be taken to gain the necessary knowledge of this). Professional medical care should be sought.

◆ HOMEOPATHIC CARE

Aconite is the first remedy to give for any acute mental shock when great fear and anxiety are seen. *Arnica* is given for any physical shock due to physical trauma, especially concussion to the head. If conscious, a person can say he is fine even when not fine or does not want to be touched. Other remedies may follow in head injury, including *Hypericum* and *Natrum sulphuricum*. *Opium* is also a remedy for extreme emotional shock and fright, and is similar to *Aconite*. Both remedies are indicated if one has witnessed a terrible accident or experienced war trauma.

Carbo veg is useful for any state of collapse with blueness of the face and difficulty breathing. People can look lifeless. There is often a need for fresh air and being fanned, even if already outside, although they may feel cold and have cold breath. The pulse may be imperceptible. General weakness from any shock is seen.

Camphor is needed in similar conditions of collapse with great icy coldness as a result of shock. Even though cold, they may not want to be covered. Both remedies are needed if someone collapses from diarrhea, along with *Arsenicum album* and *Veratrum album*.

Ignatia is the remedy for emotional shock and grief, when there is sudden bad news, loss, disappointment or grief. Emotionally there is a distraught state with sobbing and sighing, or an inability to cry, even if there is a desire to. There can be spasms and twitching of the body in the shock state and even unconsciousness, which *Aconite*, *Chamomilla* and *Coffea* also can have.

Gelsemium is also good for shock when there is confusion, sleepiness, a heaviness of the body and the eyelids feel heavy with a desire to fall asleep. There can be great anxiety and trembling remaining after the shock.

COMBINATION STRATEGY In any state of sudden collapse, you can combine *Arsenicum album*, *Camphor* and *Carbo veg* if the picture isn't clear. *Aconite* and *Opium* can be combined if there is extreme fear remaining after a shock.

Sleeplessness

Sleeplessness can be caused by many factors. Sometimes it is a chronic ongoing condition and in that case, constitutional homeopathic treatment is needed. In more acute situations, it is mostly due to anxiety, jetlag, or because of another physical condition being experienced. There are many allopathic and herbal options to help with sleep, including sleeping tablets, melatonin (if available) and various herbal and homeopathic formulas. The following homeopathic remedies are suggested for simple occasional sleeplessness. Valeriana can be taken herbally to aid sleep.

♦ HOMEOPATHIC CARE

Cocculus is a good remedy when after having missed sleep, it is difficult to relax and fall asleep. This can happen when traveling overnight or when very little sleep has been had for days. It is also excellent for states of anxiety and worry that come from the stress of travel, or looking after people and feeling overwhelmed. Often one can feel heavy, tired, dizzy and confused.

Chamomilla and *Coffea* are two other good remedies to consider. In *Chamomilla*, which is excellent for children, there is great agitation, frustration and anger. Children just cannot be pacified, nothing will relieve them. It is good to give just before sleep. In *Coffea*, there is great over excitability, restlessness and the mind feels it is working too hard. It is good when there are many things on your mind, perhaps anticipating events and simply unable to relax.

Nux vomica is also excellent and similar to *Chamomilla* and *Coffea*. There is great nervousness, irritation and even anger, a wound up, touchy state. It is the remedy to give if sleeplessness comes from drinking too much alcohol. *Ignatia* should be given when you feel you can't sleep from grief, worry and anxiety, when you feel sad and weepy and your moods are changeable and erratic.

Spinal (Back) Injury

● **GENERAL CARE**

In any injury (or pain) to the back, it is important to know how serious the injury is. It is important to keep still initially in evaluating the nature of the injury. If the injury involves a break to the back, then undue movement may lead to paralysis or at least a complication of the situation. Nerves may be involved in back injuries. If the injury seems serious, then wait until the shock has died down before moving. If less serious, still be careful. If the injury is to the coccyx, it may be broken. Seeing a doctor for a diagnosis can be very important to get an idea of the severity of the injury.

● HOMEOPATHIC CARE

Arnica is the first remedy if the injury does not seem severe and there is a simple jolt or shock to the spine, giving one tablet three times a day for two days. *Hypericum* can then be given to follow for two days. *Hypericum* is especially indicated for injuries to the coccyx when there are shooting pains and difficulty in sitting. For injuries to the neck, including whiplash, *Arnica* should first be given, followed by *Hypericum*.

Gelsemium is needed if there is residual dizziness or nausea, the head feels heavy and there is mental confusion. If that doesn't finish it, give *Cocculus*. If mental confusion remains or generally you do not feel normal, even months or years after the injury take *Natrum sulphuricum*, once daily for three days.

Rhus tox or *Ruta grav* can follow *Arnica* in injuries to the back due to straining and over lifting, especially if there is stiffness in the back with difficulty to straighten up when rising from sitting. There can be spasms of pain after injury, especially after exposure to cold and damp weather and pains are better from pressure and warmth. *Nux vomica* can follow if the spasms are not fully relieved. *Ledum* is indicated when pains from a strain move position and also come with great stiffness. However, pains are often worse from heat, the opposite of *Rhus tox*, *Ruta grav* and *Nux vomica*.

Chamomilla is good when the pains seem intolerable, forcing one from bed and pacing the floor. The pain induces a lot of anger, similar to *Nux vomica*. *Aesculus* is useful for intense back pain, making the person feel lame and unable to walk and if complicated by symptoms of piles. *See Pain section for other general pain remedies.*

Sprains

A sprain to a joint, often the ankle, knee or wrist can be debilitating and very painful initially and greatly limiting if traveling. It can also be difficult to distinguish from a break and a medical evaluation is often needed to confirm the diagnosis.

● **GENERAL CARE**

Ensure the injured part is supported well with an appropriate bandage. Follow good first aid care. Be careful to rest the part as much as possible but if it is not broken, then gradual gentle motion is good. Use topical treatment of *Arnica* cream and/or *Rhus tox* cream on the injured part. Try not to re-injure the part by using it too much. Check with a doctor to see if it is only a sprain or whether a bone may be broken if pain continues.

◆ **HOMEOPATHIC CARE**

Arnica is the first remedy to give for the basic trauma, especially if there is bruising and swelling to the area and it is worse from touch. It should then be followed by another remedy depending on the symptoms. *Bryonia* should be given when it is excruciatingly painful, and is worse for any movement, touch and jar. There is a need to keep the injured part very still.

Rhus tox is good when there is great stiffness in the injured area and pain on initial movement, but which then gets better from continued motion and also at times by warmth. *Ruta grav* is similar to *Rhus tox* and is especially indicated in injuries to wrists, tennis elbow and small joints, as well as the shin area, where the periosteum is involved. *Ledum* follows *Arnica* well when the part remains bruised and swollen, in spite of *Arnica* and especially if the injured part feels cold.

Surgery

All forms of surgery are traumatic events for the body and mind and some homeopathic remedies can be helpful in overcoming the trauma involved.

◆ HOMEOPATHIC CARE

Arnica is the first remedy to consider for any surgery, including having teeth extracted or operated on. Give one tablet three times the day before any surgery and then three times daily for up to three days after. *Bellis perennis* is to be given if surgery is on deep abdominal tissue, often leaving the person feeling very sore and bruised.

Staphysagria is good when there are lacerated wounds, due to surgical incision, especially in very sensitive areas such as the abdomen or genitalia. Often the wound feels very sensitive and there can be a feeling of violation and great oversensitivity.

Calendula can be used in a tincture and applied locally as well as in a homeopathic potency if the wound of the surgery is very painful. *(See Wounds section)*. Also look at remedies in the Shock section if there is shock involved. If the surgery required general anesthetic and the person is having a hard time recovering from this, feeling spacey and disoriented, then *Phosphorus* can be given three times daily for up to three days. If nausea remains after anesthetic, give *Arsenicum album* and follow with *Nux vomica* if that doesn't work.

Travel Sickness

Travel sickness is a common affliction but which can be very debilitating. Some people get it much worse than others and if that is the case, preventative care should be taken, both conventionally and homeopathically. If you know of a homeopathic remedy that has worked before, then this should be taken before you travel. Don't wait until you get sick!

♦ HOMEOPATHIC CARE

Tabacum is the first remedy to consider for serious travel sickness, especially sea sickness. There is often a deathly nausea, your face has a white pallor with cold perspiration and you often feel a great sinking feeling in the stomach. There can be weakness and trembling and even a feeling like you might even die. Any tobacco smoke makes symptoms worse.

Cocculus has nausea, vomiting, dizziness and weakness due to movement of a boat or car. One can't look at any moving object and the nausea is worse at the sight or smell of food. Symptoms are better when lying down and worse when sitting up and raising the head. *Nux vomica* has violent nausea, gagging and retching but you are unable to fully expel vomit.

COMBINATION STRATEGY If in doubt, take one tablet of every remedy, mixing in water and taking one tsp. every five to ten minutes until there is relief or simply take in tablet form.

Wounds

● GENERAL CARE

Any wound in which the skin is broken needs to be cleaned and protected from infection. Be very attentive of even small wounds in the tropics, especially around the feet. Clean well and cover if possible. General first aid care with use of band aids and bandages need to be used and homeopathic care used to supplement this. Carry *Calendula* tincture and tea tree oil for basic disinfectant. If a wound is deep, due to a nail or other pointed object, try and get the wound to bleed. This is to prevent tetanus which can only grow where there is no oxygen. Once a wound is dressed, it can be left for days until the wound is somewhat healed. The dressing should not be changed. Even if the wound continues to weep, do not change it daily, only when totally necessary. Spray *Calendula* tincture onto the bandage which will maintain the disinfectant of the wound. Internal homeopathic remedies can be given along with local applications. Plain sugar can also be put on a wound and then dressed with a bandage.

● HOMEOPATHIC CARE

Calendula in a homeopathic tincture can be used to wash and clean any wound, including a puncture wound, ulcer and laceration. Some tincture should be put into warm water and the injured area cleaned thoroughly. It should be followed by *Calendula* or Hyper/cal cream or ointment. It is imperative to thoroughly clean a puncture wound to prevent infection. Tea tree oil and/or lavender oil can be used topically instead of or along with the *Calendula* and *Hypericum*.

Calendula can be given in a 30c potency for lacerated wounds, especially if very painful. *Ledum* is given for punctured wounds with *Hypericum* to follow in injury to nerve rich areas with sharp shooting pains. *Staphysagria* is needed for painful lacerations, especially in vulnerable areas, e.g., abdomen, around the eyes, genitalia etc. There is a great feeling of violation, emotional sensitivity and vulnerability. *Silicea* is useful for splintered wounds, in order to help extract the splinter or spines in the skin.

Chapter Four
Emotional Conditions

If you are feeling anxious, angry or any other emotional stress, breathing slowly and deeply can help. Often we forget to do this and it can greatly relieve anxiety by using breathing to calm down. There is a type of breathing in yoga where you contract the back of the throat, narrowing the passages for air, allowing more control of both inhalation and exhalation. It is called ujjayi breath and it can greatly help when emotions of all sorts threaten to overwhelm. You can use this method to breathe slowly but deeply for a few minutes but the main thing is to use the breath to calm down and to gain control of strong emotions.

Strong emotional feelings can come up at any time and for many reasons and in homeopathy it can be an important part of understanding what remedy may be useful, both for physical conditions and also to deal with intense emotional states that may arise, whether traveling or simply in one's daily life.

Anger

Anger that exists out of proportion to a situation is something to be very aware of. In cultures where anger is not appropriate or when faced with situations that are very stressful, one has to cultivate great restraint. Homeopathic treatment should be given if this is a common occurrence or when there are physical and/or emotional consequences from becoming angry. If anger is a common reaction to situations, then constitutional homeopathic care or some form of therapy should be taken.

● HOMEOPATHIC CARE

Colocynthis and *Staphysagria* are needed if anger comes after an experience of being humiliated or treated badly and one feels indignant, frustrated and unable to express these feelings. With *Staphysagria*, one feels oversensitive, even weepy, and often very humiliated. Anger may not be felt, one feels simply upset, or one can feel a great anger with a desire to throw things or break things. There is great frustration. In *Colocynthis*, similar feelings are also experienced, often along with great cramping, especially in the abdomen, the pains doubling one up and there is a need to press deeply into the abdomen for relief. With both remedies, the initial anger is suppressed and then other symptoms arise, both physical and psychological. Anger may come up later, along with great indignation. Anger can be initially stronger with *Colocynthis*.

Nux vomica is needed if there are feelings of pent up wrath, feeling extremely touchy and sensitive to all impressions, including noises, smells etc. One feels intolerant and impatient and it takes a lot of energy to contain the anger.

Chamomilla is needed when capriciousness and rage are felt and one just doesn't know what to do. There is frustration, touchiness, impatience and intolerantce but not so full of rage as when *Nux vomica* is needed. *Chamomilla* is great for angry children who throw everything they are given and cannot be placated in anyway.

Anxiety

Anxiety exists for many reasons and may often be utterly appropriate to the situation. Anticipatory anxiety is also common when traveling or before exams. It should not be treated unless it does not go away or seems extreme for the situation at hand.

● HOMEOPATHIC CARE

Aconite is the first remedy to consider if anxiety is felt as a result of an extreme shock or fright. If a deep shock is experienced, even as extreme as feeling as if one could die, e.g., being in or even watching an accident, then *Aconite* is the remedy.

Gelsemium is the remedy if one feels more anticipatory anxiety or a shock which makes one tremble and very apprehensive, as if on is going to experience the same thing again. It is the first remedy for all kinds of anticipatory anxiety, even to having diarrhea. This is a great remedy to have for all kinds of travel based anxiety.

Coffea is needed if there is anxiety as if one is wired up on coffee and oversensitive to everything, including noises, smells and any stimulus. This is an example of how homeopathy works. Like Cures Like. *Coffea* is an excellent remedy for anxiety states, especially when one is very tense, agitated or impatient and the mind is racing very fast.

🍃 HERBAL CARE

Valeriana can be taken for nervous anxiety and sleeplessness. *Rescue remedy* (A Bach Flower Remedy) can also be taken for any kind of shock and anxiety. It can be used along with a homeopathic remedy and you can take it as often as feels needed when anxiety arises.

Fright

Acute fright can be experienced at any time. Unpredictable events can occur at any time and the shock involved can leave a lasting effect. *See Chapter Three: Accidents, Injuries and Trauma, Shock section and also Anxiety above.*

⬤ GENERAL CARE

If you experience or see a person experiencing a fright do nothing until you feel the shock diminish. Sit down and breathe deeply. If the fright continues then take one of the homeopathic remedies.

🔻 HOMEOPATHIC CARE

Aconite and *Gelsemium* are the two main remedies to consider, similar to anxiety, and their symptom picture is described above in the anxiety section and elsewhere. Both *Gelsemium* and *Aconite* are good after experiencing an earthquake or similar type of trauma.

Stramonium is a very good remedy for ailments from fright when great fear and terror remain, and also has a strong fear of the dark, of being alone at night and of dogs. It is one of the main remedies when extreme fear is due to any violence seen or experienced.

Opium is needed when great fear remains after experiencing or witnessing a terrible event, e.g., accident, war trauma etc. In *Opium* one feels as if frozen in the fear, a 'fear of fear' and the only escape is to become emotionally numb, and cut off from your feelings.

Cocculus is needed if one feels weak, dizzy and dull after a fright. There is great heaviness and similar to *Gelsemium*, the head can feel too heavy to hold up. One can also take *Rescue Remedy*, 3 drops, every 15-60 minutes until you feel relief. Take it as necessary along with a homeopathic remedy.

Grief

Grief is a normal reaction to emotional trauma but at times it is hard to overcome. Taking homeopathic remedies is useful to help any state of grief.

◆ HOMEOPATHIC CARE

Ignatia is the first remedy to think of for any grief, be it romantic loss, or the death of a close friend or family member. The feeling is one of shock and an inability to reconcile the grief. Emotionally one often feels as if to cry but can't, or can't stop crying. Sobbing may be uncontrollable with much sighing and even cramping in parts of the body. There may be a lump in the throat and a choking feeling, making it difficult to swallow. Moods are changing all the time.

Natrum muriaticum often follows *Ignatia* and is needed when there is a feeling of sadness and grief but with no weeping. One may want to weep but simply can't express feelings. Everything is held in. There s a desire to be alone and think of the grief, but that doesn't help. Listening to sad music makes the sadness worse but sharing it with people also doesn't help.

Cocculus is needed when there is great sadness, heaviness and weakness. One may be unable to sleep at night and in the day one feels dazed and unable to focus on anything else, as if in another world. *Gelsemium* is also similar.

Pulsatilla is needed if one feels deserted, forsaken and lost. There is much weepiness and unable to control emotions. Moods change all the time and there is a great desire for company and consolation, or a feeling to be alone and then later really wanting to be in company. Moods are very changeable.

Chapter Five
Digestive Conditions

Abdominal Pain

It is important to know if abdominal problems, especially pain which is very intense, could be due to appendicitis, pelvic inflammatory disease, menstrual problems, gall bladder problems, inflammation of the pancreas or spleen, liver problems or obstruction of the intestines. Some pain can also be referred from the back, perhaps due to kidney problems or structural back problems. If pain persists, see a medical practitioner for a diagnosis.

See Constipation, Diarrhea, Dysentery, Food poisoning, Heartburn, Hepatitis, Indigestion sections.

Appendicitis

Appendicitis is an inflammation of the appendix, a small protrusion found in the small intestine. Appendicitis often requires surgery because if the appendix bursts, it can lead to a more generalized infection of the whole body (peritonitis), which can be life threatening. It is very important to get a medical diagnosis if there is any doubt about any abdominal pain. It is not always easy to diagnose. The classic area of pain is in the right lower half of the abdomen, two to three inches in from the hip joint. Pain is often better when pressure is applied but then gets much worse when pressure is released suddenly. Sometimes, pain can initially be felt more in the navel (umbilical) region and radiates from there. If pain begins there for no apparent reason and doesn't go away in 24 hours, press into the appendix region to see if there is any sensitivity there. If in doubt, get a medical diagnosis.

● **GENERAL CARE**

As with any inflammation, drink more water. Do not do any strenuous exertions. Relax and rest. Do not eat anything for 24 hours and see if that makes a difference. If in doubt, take one of the homeopathic remedies and head for the nearest emergency room hospital.

◆ **HOMEOPATHIC CARE**

Bryonia is the first remedy to consider for appendicitis. One may experience an intense pain either in the lower right quadrant of the abdomen or in the umbilical area and any movement makes the pain worse. One wants to keep very still. Putting pressure on the painful area may make the pain better and any jarring makes it worse.

Belladonna is the second remedy to think of, especially if the pain comes on very suddenly and intensely, the pain being bursting, sharp and/or throbbing. There may be a high, burning fever, which is higher and more intense than felt in the *Bryonia* picture. With both remedies there may be increased thirst.

Arnica may also be needed if there is a bruised, sore feeling in the appendix region and one doesn't want the area touched, but *Bryonia* should be given first and if necessary followed by one of the other remedies. If the remedy is correct, a change should be seen within one to three hours. The remedy should be taken ideally in liquid, one tsp. every five to ten minutes.

✐ HERBAL CARE

Take *Echinacea* tincture, 30 drops, hourly for one day.

Colic

Colic is a painful contraction of parts of the body, most often felt in the abdomen (intestines) and also in the kidneys and ureters (tubes from the kidney to bladder) and the bile duct near the liver. Abdominal colic is often seen in young babies and children when they are having difficulty digesting milk or food. Symptoms are extremely painful contractions of the affected part, making the person double up in pain and the pain comes in spasms. Often you want to grab the painful part and keep it still or put much pressure onto it.

See Chapter Six : Common conditions: Cystitis and Kidney Disease. Also see Chapter Three: Accidents and Injuries, Pain section.

● GENERAL CARE

It is good to allow the person to lie down in whichever position they want and just give support. Having this type of pain can be very unsettling. If it is kidney colic, it may indicate stones in the kidney and urinary tract which may require medical intervention.

● HOMEOPATHIC CARE

Colocynthis is the first remedy to consider for abdominal colic. The pain feels as if the abdomen is twisting and cutting, or being squeezed between two stones. There can be great restlessness and wanting to bend double and to press very intensely into the abdomen. It can also be indicated in colic of the kidneys. It is excellent when colic comes after a bout of anger or indignation, similar to that of *Staphysagria*. If anger is the precipitating cause and *Colocynthis* doesn't work, give *Staphysagria*.

Chamomilla is the first remedy to consider for colic in babies, when there is much screaming and weeping and the child wants to be carried all the time.

Nux vomica is a good remedy for all sorts of colic, intestinal as well as kidney and liver, especially if from over indulging in rich food or alcohol. There can be great irritability with the symptoms.

Bryonia is good when there is a desire to stay very still with the pains. Every movement makes it worse and keeping still is the best thing to do.

Berberis is useful particularly in kidney (renal) colic, especially when the pain is spreading out in waves to the rest of the body from the kidney region.

Magnesium phosphoricum can be given if *Colocynthis* is indicated but doesn't work or where the symptoms are much better from warm or hot applications to the abdomen as well as bending double.

Lycopodium has colic associated with liver and gall bladder issues, often seen with abdominal swelling and much gas being passed. There is a great aversion to clothing around the waist. It can be given in kidney colic when the right kidney is affected.

Constipation

This can be due to many reasons. It is important to investigate any possible mechanical causes for constipation, especially in young children. Hemorrhoids may also be a cause of constipation. Mostly, constipation is a chronic condition that requires more constitutional treatment. However, when 'on the road' constipation can be a frequent problem, due to dietary differences and also due to being unable or reluctant to go in strange places. One should seek medical attention if the constipation persists for more than five days without any bowel movement or is associated with much rectal bleeding, weight loss or frequent intense pain in the intestines.

● GENERAL CARE

Keep hydrated. Drink enough water, wherever you are. If you need to make a rehydration mixture, use one teaspoon of salt with eight teaspoons of sugar and one liter of clean water. Eat food that encourages bowel function – fresh fruit, vegetables, and especially prunes or figs. Ensure you get enough roughage in your diet, and ideally whole grains. Avoid too much white rice.

● HOMEOPATHIC CARE

Nux vomica is the best remedy to take for simple constipation on the road. There can be frequent urging but very little or nothing comes out. This may also be associated with painful hemorrhoids. One can feel quite irritable with the constipation and a feeling of being unfinished after a stool.

Bryonia can also be given when the stool seems very dry and there is a general dryness of the whole body, especially the mouth and lips.

● HERBAL CARE

Take probiotics with you when you travel to help maintain a healthy flora in your intestines. Ground flax seeds or Chia seeds can be used and also psyllium is very useful for constipation as well as diarrhea. *See Diarrhea section.*

Diaper (Nappy) Rash

This is a condition where there is inflammation around the anus, leading to redness and at times rawness, pain and great discomfort. it can become infected, mainly due to bacteria or fungus.

● GENERAL CARE

Allow the area to be open to the air as much as possible. Ensure diapers are changed frequently. Wash the area thoroughly and dry very well. Use a good cream, such as homeopathic *Calendula* cream (especially if more infected) or baby powder. Breast milk can be used as well.

♦ HOMEOPATHIC CARE

Belladonna is needed when the child's anus is very red with great burning and a fever is involved.

Chamomilla is the remedy when the child is screaming inconsolably and it feels nothing gives relief give.

Rhus tox is excellent when there are weeping blisters and great redness with restlessness.

● HERBAL CARE

Use *Calendula* cream.

Diarrhea

Diarrhea is one of the most frequent experiences of travelers. Often due to eating bad food or water and/or infections with viruses, bacteria or amoebas, diarrhea is the natural reaction of the body to purge the offending bugs. Suppressing diarrhea should only be done when absolutely necessary and should not be a routine event when diarrhea ensues. Antibiotics such as Cipro should not be given in the first few days of diarrhea before it is known what type of diarrhea one has. Use natural methods first. While most cases of diarrhea are self-limiting (up to 80% clear up on their own in three days) some can become more serious conditions and need to be treated effectively. Do not immediately take drugs to bung you up (Imodium, Lomotil etc.) if you get a dose of diarrhea. Let nature take its course unless you have to travel and could find yourself in trouble. Normally the body has to purge the toxins from the system. Taking these medications simply prevents your body doing what it needs to do. They can also cause complications if you have dysentery or have any blood in your stool. Also do not give them to children. Give some rehydration salts/powders and wait it out.

If taking conventional drugs, ensure they are what they say they are and are safe. Many drugs found in the developing world can be unsafe, or have been banned in other countries. Seek appropriate medical advice for diagnosis and treatment. Any lingering diarrhea that continues after travel has to be checked out by a medical specialist for diagnostic purposes. Do not ignore lingering symptoms, especially after travel to 'exotic' places.

One of the most common infections is giardia, a protozoa which can be easily caught both in tropical and temperate climates. It is less acute than other infectious diarrheas but tends to last much longer, often with weakness, fullness and very offensive fatty stools. At times it only begins once back from a vacation due to an incubation period of over one week. Having a stool test can be useful to confirm diagnosis. However, homeopathic treatment should be commenced immediately. The most specific remedy for it is *China*. Also *See Dysentery section*. Treatment should be given for at least one week. Be patient. Improvement will begin between one to three days but will take longer to fully get better. The remedy should be taken three times a day. It is also the remedy for amoebiasis when one generally feels weak, bloated, lacking appetie and perhaps some diarrhea of constipation. It can be quite mild, with general lethargy or more severe with real weakness, much offensive gas and stool. Avoid eating fruit, dairy and meat.

Cholera is historically one of the most intense and dangerous diarrheal diseases but today, for most travelers and in developed societies, it is rarely seen. It occurs most commonly in times and places where hygiene and clean water is severely lacking and many people are living together in cramped circumstances, e.g., war situations and other natural traumas. It is a bacterial disease and is spread through contaminated water and food. Some people can be carriers of the disease and once infected, the incubation period is normally between two to seven days.
See Chapter Eight: Tropical Conditions: Cholera.

Diarrhea can also be associated with other conditions, including malaria and typhoid. If diarrhea comes with a fever, consider these conditions. If there is fever and blood in the stool, consider bacillary dysentery, but if there's blood in the stool with no fever, it may be amoebic dysentery. Bilharzia/Schistosomiaisis may also have blood in stool and also urine with no fever. If diarrhea is extremely severe, like rice water, but no blood is seen and no fever, consider cholera.

Liver flukes may be another reason for diarrhea, often associated in the acute phase with nausea and abdominal pain. More long term symptoms include fatigue, weight loss, abdominal discomfort, jaundice and anorexia. They can affect liver and bile duct function and other more chronic conditions can ensue. They are often caught from eating undercooked fish and are particularly prevalent in Far East Asia. It can be tested for and conventional treatment is available.

● **GENERAL CARE**

As a prevention, ensure the food you eat is well cooked, especially meat. Drink only water that has been well boiled and purified or use bottled water. *See Chapter Two: Being Prepared, Food and Water section.*

Once you have diarrhea, avoid milk, meat, fatty, spicy and any other irritating foods. Keep to a simple diet or simply do not eat for 24-48 hours. Bananas are OK but avoid citrus fruit. If you feel hungry, plain white rice with a little plain yoghurt is good or just rice and other dry foods – bread, toast, etc. Keep hydrated by drinking good water and if dehydration is suspected, introduce some re-hydration ingredients with the water.

Tea made from neem and artemisia leaves may relieve diarrhea and also tea from leaves of the guava and mango tree can be effective (1 tablespoon of pounded leaves each). The latter can be mixed together and is good for amoebic dysentery. Fruit should be avoided but eating ripe mangoes can help in amoebic dysentery.

◆ HOMEOPATHIC CARE

Arsenicum album. is the first remedy to consider in acute diarrhea of all sorts. It is excellent for all food poisoning. Diarrhea can be very acute, with great burning when passing stool and when nausea and vomiting comes with it. Often there is exhaustion after passing stool, feeling worse at the sight or smell of food and often feeling chilled.

Veratrum album often looks like *Arsenicum album*, with nausea and/or vomiting along with the diarrhea, but it has more chill and cold perspiration with the stool, especially on the forehead.

Podophyllum has very characteristic rumbling and gurgling in the abdomen, often just before stool, which then comes out in a violent intense, explosive gush. There can also be involuntary stool, especially at night. The stool can be either very odorous or doesn't smell at all.

Colocynthis is indicated if diarrhea is experienced with intense cramping pains in the abdomen. It feels as if the intestines are being twisted or squeezed and the pain forces one to bend double and/or to press intensely into the abdomen.

Nux vomica also can have intense cramping, often just before stool, and the urging is intense and nearly always unsatisfying. There can also be spasmodic nausea, retching and vomiting, which again doesn't relieve. *Nux vomica* and *Arsenicum album* are mostly the two remedies needed for acute food poisoning. With both remedies one can feel very chilly and need to be covered.

Aloe is a good remedy for travelers' diarrhea. In this remedy there is a feeling of great insecurity, specifically in the bowels. It feels as if one could lose stool at any moment. When passing wind, the feeling is as if one could lose stool so always having to be near the toilet. There can be a lot of loud flatus with the stool and it is sputtering and/or hot. There can be pain in the back with the stool. Emotionally, one can feel very insecure, being in unfamiliar places and feeling out of control with the situation.

Chamomilla is a great remedy for children's diarrhea. It looks like chopped eggs and spinach and has a rotten, offensive odor, like bad eggs. The diarrhea often comes with cramping colic and great peevishness. It is a remedy for diarrhea while teething.

Gelsemium is good when diarrhea is due totally to an anticipatory anxiety before an event of some sort. *See Chapter Four: Emotional Conditions, Anxiety section.*

COMBINATION STRATEGY If in doubt which remedy to give, mix one tablet of *Arsenicum album*, *Podophyllum* and *Veratrum album* together in two to four ounces of water and take one tsp. every one to three hours until change, depending on the severity of symptoms.

🍃 HERBAL CARE

Goldenseal tincture can be taken for most forms of diarrhea, especially by E coli infection but it should not to be taken in pregnant or breast feeding women, or taken for longer than two weeks. Ispaghula (named Fybogel or Isogel in the UK) or Isabgol or more commonly known as psyllium can be taken for both diarrhea and constipation. It originates from the plantago family and is used to bulk up food, aiding peristaltic action in constipation. In diarrhea it helps absorb liquid in the small intestine. It needs to be taken with enough water or it can have a choking effect as it becomes sticky very quickly. Medicinal charcoal can be taken for mild diarrhea (one tablespoon three times daily for two days). Ensure the charcoal is sterile through heating and the wood used is not poisonous. Grapefruit seed extract can be used as well.

Dysentery

Dysentery is a diarrhea mostly caused by amoebas or bacillus although initially it can be treated like any other type of diarrhea. Most diarrheas of travelers are not dysentery, but if symptoms don't clear up or get better after three days, it should be considered as it indicates that parasites or bacillus (Shigellosis) are involved. If it is amoebic dysentery, it can continue for a long time, beyond three weeks when more serious. In both situations there is often blood with the stool and much mucous and undigested food. With both amoebic and bacillary dysentery it is important to treat effectively, especially when traveling. It can lead to great depletion, weakness, dehydration, secondary liver problems (abscesses), eye problems, arthritis etc. It is useful to get a medical diagnosis of what type of dysentery it is. Both types are spread mostly through food and water, though flies can transmit the disease.

Bacillary dysentery may begin more suddenly in more serious cases, often with a fever (whereas amoebic dysentery often has no fever) and there can be severe cramping in the abdomen. Stools are very frequent, explosive, with much mucus, blood, watery and frothy diarrhea. It is often odorless. Cases may be mild and recover within a few days or may continue for up to three weeks. However, even when symptoms have disappeared, one can carry and spread the condition for some months.

Amoebic dysentery tends to start more slowly but then develops into more frequent copious stools than found in bacillary dysentery. Often one does not feel particularly unwell at this stage, in contrast to bacillary dysentery. It can be found both in temperate and tropical zones. Its severity is often dependent on the overall health of the person. Healthy people can catch this and have very mild symptoms which soon disappear. However, it can become a more chronic condition with intermittent symptoms of loose stool and also constipation which continues even for years. It will be aggravated by other factors such as diet, exhaustion and other diseases. If symptoms are more extreme and acute, the onset is sudden with frequent urging of offensive watery, mucus laden stools, which are very offensive. Stools may be involuntary, and there can be cramping and spasms in the rectum. In some cases, the amoebas reach the liver, with symptoms of fullness in the liver region (right upper quadrant of the abdomen, below the ribs), pain referred to the right shoulder, fever with sweating and loss of appetite and weight. Loss of weight and appetite can occur in any of the above situations.

In more serious cases, if symptoms do not get better within one week, then professional homeopathic care or other medical intervention should be sought.

● GENERAL CARE

Prevention is key through effective hygiene. Always wash your hands, especially after stool. Avoid bad food and water. Do not touch things unnecessarily. Be careful being around others as you can still spread the condition even when feeling better. Keep hydrated at all times. Do not eat food that aggravates the digestive system. Avoid spicy, creamy, rich foods and fruit. Keep the diet very minimal; plain rice, bananas, and other simple foods if the symptoms are severe. Yoghurt is OK as it helps replenish the bowel flora but it may not be digested too easily, so eat only small amounts. Conventional care involves appropriate antibiotics for bacillary dysentery and often Metronidazole (Flagyl) or Tinidazole for amoebic dysentery. Flagyl is also often given for giardia, but it can affect some people adversely and may not totally clear up the condition. It should be taken more as a last resort and natural methods tried first.

◆ HOMEOPATHIC CARE

China is the main remedy to consider, especially if there is great bloating and fullness in the abdomen. One can feel very exhausted, depleted and weak, which is much worse after stool and often with ittle appetite, feeling full after a few bites. Stool may be bloody and with mucus, and diarrhea may alternate with constipation. Passing gas doesn't relieve the bloating and the liver may also feel full and hard. It is often needed when the symptoms have become more chronic and long term. Initially diarrhea may be much worse after fruit and/or rich food. It is the main remedy for giardia.

Mercurius (vivus or solubulis) is one of the best remedies to take for more acute dysentery, (both amoebic and bacillary). There is frequent painful urging of bloody stool and there is very little relief after stool. The urging can be painful and fairly constant. Often the stool is very offensive, even metallic smelling and also perspiration can be offensive. One feels very 'toxic'. Fever is often present, but not too high. Perspiration is seen with fever, which can feel oily. There can be fullness in the liver region and great weakness and depletion. If there is much blood with the stool and a constant, ineffectual urging and unsatisfied feeling, then *Mercurius corrosivus* (another form of mercury) should be taken if *Mercurius* does not fully cure.

Baptisia is indicated in more serious states, when there is great exhaustion, depletion and achiness in the body. Stools are dark, thin, bloody and offensive. There is distension and rumbling and mentally very low, confused, tired and tending to fall asleep very easily, even when being spoken to. The face can look besotted and there is an ongoing low fever. *Arnica* can also be taken if it looks like *Baptisia* and it hasn't worked and there is soreness and aching in the body and the bed feels hard when lying down.

Sulphur is very useful in more chronic situations when the stool is very offensive, burning, bloody and with mucus. There may be great urging on waking in the morning. The rectum may burn intensely after stool and flatus can be very offensive. *Sulphur* should be given if you have tried other remedies which either haven't worked or only worked partially. All the remedies listed in the diarrhea section can also be thought of.

COMBINATION STRATEGY If no remedy is clear mix one tablet of *Baptisia*, *China* and *Mercurius* in two to four ounces of water and take one tsp. three to six times a day, depending on severity of symptoms.

⊘ **HERBAL CARE**
Take charcoal tablets and/or clay internally.

Food Poisoning

Food poisoning can happen at any time and in any place. It is often experienced traveling due to dirty food and water, yet it can occur equally when at home or eating at a restaurant. One of the most common causes is salmonella bacteria and other bacteria and also some viruses. Symptoms tend to come on very suddenly and intensely and also often diminish within one to three days.

● GENERAL CARE

If possible, keep fluid intake up but do not worry too much at the beginning. Endure the acute symptoms until you feel some improvement. Do not eat anything until vomiting and acute diarrhea have decreased significantly.

● HOMEOPATHIC CARE

Arsenicum album is the first remedy to take for simple food poisoning. There is sudden intense diarrhea and nausea and vomiting, which can all come on at the same time. Nausea is often worse at the sight or smell of food. *Veratrum album* has very similar symptoms but has more cold perspiration, especially on the forehead. Both have weakness and prostration after stool.

Nux vomica is the next remedy to take, especially when there is great cramping in the abdomen and violent retching and vomiting, with the feeling that one just can't bring everything up. Spasms can be felt anywhere in the body and nausea is much worse from the smell of food.

Podophyllum is useful when there is a lot of bloating, rumbling and gurgling in the intestines followed by a violent, forcible stool exploding from the rectum. There may also be cramping in the abdomen before stool. *See Diarrhea section.*

Hemorrhoids

Hemorrhoids (piles) are due to enlarged varicose veins in the rectal area. They can come as a consequence of constipation, and some people are more predisposed to them than others. Recurrent pain and distress in the rectal area should be examined for its causation, as often such symptoms are simply put down to hemorrhoids when other factors may be at play. Piles may be internal or external or may be exposed only after straining at stool. Once piles have become chronic and seriously engorged, surgery can be required. However, homeopathic remedies can be very helpful in earlier stages. Constitutional treatment is usually the most effective approach to this condition.

● HOMEOPATHIC CARE

Nux vomica is the first remedy to consider for very sensitive, painful piles, especially due to overstraining when passing stool. The pain can be very intense and sharp and worse for any touch.

Aloe also has piles from constipation which protrude and there is a great sense of pressure forcing downwards, creating insecurity in the region, as if stool can be lost, even if no diarrhea is there. There can be bleeding from the rectum and much wind.

Aesculus is one of the main remedies for piles, with or without constipation. The main symptom is a sensation of sticks in the rectum and sharp pains extending up the back. There is a feeling of great congestion, fullness and burning in the rectum and the back can feel as if it is giving out.

Sulphur is thought of if there is great heat and burning in the rectal area. If very sensitive piles are found along with cracks in the skin around the rectum, then *Nitric acid* can be given.

COMBINATION STRATEGY It may not be able to easily identify one remedy for this condition. If so, then mix one tablet of each remedy that seems indicated into four ounces of water and give one sip/tsp. three times daily for three days. Some relief should be seen by then.

Hepatitis

Hepatitis is an infection of the liver. There are three main types of hepatitis, termed A, B and C. Hepatitis A is the most common infection, occurring through contaminated water and is common in many developing countries. Hepatitis B and C are communicated through blood and symptoms can remain dormant for many years. In this case, we are only dealing with hepatitis A. There are two types of conventional prophylaxis for Hepatitis A, a human immunoglobulin injection and a vaccination. The former gives immunity for about four months while the latter will give a long lasting immunity. If you have previously had hepatitis A, you will normally have lifelong immunity to the disease.

Symptoms of Hepatitis A develop between two and four weeks after initial infection and often begin with symptoms similar to the 'flu. There may be fever, general malaise and weakness, aching of the body, a slightly raised temperature and a great lack of appetite, often with nausea and vomiting. There may be a strong aversion to fatty food and alcohol. There may also be diarrhea and or constipation. More characteristic, if seen, is a tenderness in the right upper abdominal region (right quadrant), where the liver is found. The area may be tender to touch and to clothing as well as to any motion. Symptoms of jaundice may be seen in many but not all cases. When this occurs, the urine becomes dark yellow and the skin and eyes become yellow.

Acute symptoms last on average two to three weeks but if more serious or the person is already weak, then overall weakness and digestive problems can last much longer. However, most cases should resolve completely within two months. However, there can be relapses after this phase, especially if a person resorts to eating as before, increasing pressure on the liver. Appropriate medical care should be taken and the person needs to live a simple, relaxed lifestyle until full recovery has been made.

In cases of hepatitis with jaundice, other diseases such as malaria and yellow fever must also be considered.

Hepatitis B and C are transmissible through blood contamination, e.g., unprotected sex, sharing needles, even having dental treatment abroad or getting tattoos. Infection can remain dormant for up to 20-30 years. Around 20% of people will develop some symptoms and in a small percentage of cases, serious liver damage can occur. Initial symptoms can be similar to Hepatitis A and diagnosis is necessary to distinguish which type of Hepatitis it is. At other times, there is no acute phase of symptoms and more chronic liver problems are the first sign.

● GENERAL CARE

General rest is crucial. There may be much weakness, along with digestive issues, so it is imperative that the person is well looked after and ideally stays in one place. Clean water and clean simple food are important. No fats, rich food, meat, alcohol, drugs or any kind of stimulants should be taken for a minimum of two months. Fruit is OK, especially papaya if in the tropics. Full recovery may take longer than two months if serious and a simple diet will need to be sustained for quite some time.

◆ HOMEOPATHIC CARE

There are a number of remedies for hepatitis in its various stages and in the acute phase, remedies may be given for the fever and other symptoms. *See Chapter Six: Common conditions, Fever and Influenza.*

China is one of the main remedies for liver problems as well as for other digestive conditions. There is often great weakness along with abdominal bloating and a very low appetite. The least food fills one up, even a few mouthfuls, and bloats the stomach. Jaundice may or may not be there. There may be diarrhea or constipation and often much gas which doesn't give any relief. There can be fever, with great weakness and easy perspiration and often an aversion to fat and rich food, and fruit can cause diarrhea.

Nux vomica is needed when there is great irritability and weakness and sensitivity to all odors and noises and one can have great nausea with retching. This is made worse from eating or drinking and even the smell of food. There is often a great aversion to fatty, rich food and alcohol. There can be sensitivity in the liver area and initially often a great chill and coldness.

Chelidonium is one of the most important liver remedies in homeopathy. There is often a specific pain in the right upper quadrant of the abdomen, but which extends through the body to the back and/or up the back to lower right shoulder blade. There can be abdominal sensitivity and bloating and some increased irritability and weakness, especially in the afternoon.

Lycopodium is very similar to *Chelidonium* and one of the great remedies for all liver problems. There is pain in the liver, often extending to the back, like *Chelidonium*, and with the pain there is great bloating of the abdomen, with much gas being passed. There is often an aversion to clothing around the waist. There can be great hunger but with fullness after a few mouthfuls, similar to *China*. There can be swelling of the liver. Symptoms can often feel worse between four to eight pm., and there is weakness and irritability on waking in the morning. *Lycopodium* is useful for chronic complications from hepatitis, even years after the initial infection.

Phosphorus is often indicated when jaundice becomes more chronic and doesn't go away, or when jaundice is present without hepatitis infection. In acute hepatitis, *Phosphorus* is indicated if there is much craving for cold water, which is often vomited when it becomes warm in the stomach.

COMBINATION STRATEGY It is good to give a homeopathic remedy and also a herbal remedy to support the liver at the same time, even if it is the same remedy, one in a homeopathic dose, the other herbal. Also, one remedy may be needed in the beginning and then another remedy may follow as the picture changes. Pay attention to the symptom picture. In acute hepatitis, give the remedy in water, taking one sip 3-5 times daily for at least one week. In more chronic cases, take one tablet daily for up to 2-4 weeks.

🖉 HERBAL CARE

Carduus mariannus (St. Mary's Thistle) tincture. Take as instructed for one to three weeks. This is both a homeopathic and herbal medicine, which can be taken to support the liver and spleen during hepatitis. It can be taken along with other homeopathic remedies.

Chelidonium (Greater Celandine) tincture can be taken in the same way as *Carduus mariannus* and is a good support for the liver. Milk thistle tincture is another excellent liver support remedy as is dandelion root.

Hiccough

Having a hiccough is a common enough condition, which seems to come on spontaneously. It may be related to how food and drink have been taken or by certain emotions and at times it can become a prolonged and debilitating condition. It is common in infants. In adults there are many solutions suggested, from drinking water upside down when bending down, breathing fast or slow or breathing into a paper bag etc.

◆ HOMEOPATHIC CARE

Ignatia is the first remedy to consider when hiccoughs come from being disappointed or any other emotional cause. *Nux vomica* is more indicated if anger precipitated the hiccoughs and where they are particularly violent in nature. *Arsenicum album* may be good if the hiccoughs came on just after taking a cold drink or during a chill or fever.

Indigestion

This can be used as a catch-all phrase for upset stomach, including heartburn and can be caused by bad food, too much food and emotional anxiety. Many times, this is not a limited acute situation but reveals an underlying vulnerability in the digestive area. However, when there is any case of simple indigestion, it can be unpleasant and can lead to further problems, like Irritable Bowel Syndrome (IBS). *See Diarrhea section.*

● GENERAL CARE

It is important to eat simple food if having any indigestion. Fatty, rich food, meat, fish and dairy products should be avoided. Acidic fruit and alcohol also should be avoided. Simple food should be taken. Papaya is excellent for indigestion. Ideally sap from a raw papaya can be taken, a few drops, mixed with some water.

See Chapter Nine: Homeopathic and Herbal Remedy list, Herbal and Plant remedies, Papaya section.

● HOMEOPATHIC CARE

Arsenicum album has the characteristic nausea, and vomiting and also diarrhea. If it is only a burning in the stomach along with just nausea, *Arsenicum album* is the first remedy to consider.

Carbo vegetabalis and *China* should be considered if bloating, tiredness, weakness and much eructation and gas are experienced. *Carbo vegetabalis* is made from vegetable charcoal and is excellent for simple indigestion, especially from eating too much rich food, fruit and ice cream. There is often weakness with distension of the abdomen. There may be lots of wind, with loud and at times rancid burps or much flatulence. All food seems to just turn to gas and clothing around the waist seems too tight. *China* has been well described in the dysentery and hepatitis sections.

Colocynthis and *Nux vomica* are two important remedies to consider especially when cramping pains are a key symptom. *Nux vomica* in particular is one of the most important remedies for indigestion that comes from simply eating too much food or too much rich, spicy food or too much alcohol. One can experience nausea and retching, a strong ineffectual urging to vomit and/or to pass stool. The stomach can feel very acidic with bitterness in the mouth and increased general irritability. *Colocynthis* is described in the diarrhea section.

Pulsatilla is a good remedy for any effects of eating too much rich food, ice cream and bad fruit and where there is a feeling of a stone in the stomach after eating. There can be regurgitations tasting of food.

Sulphur is needed if with indigestion, there are burning pains and eructations smelling or tasting like eggs. There can be great hunger, especially at 11am which comes with a sinking, weak feeling.

Nausea

There are many reasons why nausea occurs. Finding the correct homeopathic remedy depends on the reasons why the nausea is happening. Remedies are suggested partly according to the cause of the nausea and partly on the actual symptoms being experienced. The following conditions are common reasons for nausea and remedies will be found in the appropriate sections of the book: Anxiety, Cholera, Diarrhea, Fever, Food poisoning, Hangover, Indigestion, Kidney colic, Malaria, Poisonings, Pregnancy, Shock, Travel sickness, Typhoid etc.

● HOMEOPATHIC CARE

A few of the most important remedies for nausea, and when found indicated in many different conditions are *Arsenicum album*, *Cocculus*, *Ipecac*, *Nux vomica*, *Sepia*, *Tabacum* and *Veratrum album*. For basic descriptions of remedies for nausea, *see Food Poisoning and Travel Sickness sections*.

Worms

There are three main types of intestinal worms that one can catch while traveling or at home. Worm infections are very common in warmer climes and when hygiene is not so good and can affect very many people. In some people, there are little or no symptoms, while in others, symptoms are stronger. Also the type of worm affects the type of symptoms. Conventional and homeopathic treatment may be undertaken to treat them.

Good hygiene and avoiding eating undercooked meat and unwashed uncooked vegetables are key factors in not getting worms.

1. Threadworms or Pinworms. These are the common type of worm often found in children. They are small thin worms, which are often found in the stool and the anus. They create great itching in the anus, especially at night and may also lead to itching in other parts of the body. It can lead to a general restlessness, irritability and loss of appetite and weight. In adults, it may be seen simply as an intense itching anus, worse at night. Worms may or may not be seen. Children often produce more symptoms, including mood changes, irritability and loss of appetite and weight.

2. Roundworms (Ascariasis). These are very common worms found in most parts of the world. Infection happens through ingesting eggs often found in raw vegetables. There may be no symptoms or signs of worms in the stool, anus or in vomit and in the nostrils. Some children, especially in developing countries may have serious infections, leading to malnutrition, with nausea, vomiting and diarrhea. Infection may even go to the liver, with symptoms of jaundice and may infect the lungs, with symptoms of cough, difficult respiration, fever etc.

3. Tapeworms. A tapeworm is a thin, long worm that can grow considerably in the intestine. It is often symptomless, or there

may be some irritation in the anus region. Infection happens through eating raw or undercooked beef. Other types of tapeworms can be caught through eating raw or undercooked fish or in food contaminated with mouse droppings.

● GENERAL CARE

There are a number of ways to help purge worms from the system using natural methods. Some may work better than others. It is worth trying before using toxic drugs. Fasting or doing juice fasts for up to ten days can be effective, especially for pin worms. For round and tape worms, it is also important to purge the worms. Take one tablespoon of fresh coconut and then take about 50ml of castor oil mixed with around 300 ml of milk three hours later. (A non-dairy milk can be used). Repeat daily as needed. Or, take a teaspoon of powdered papaya seeds and mix with one cup of water and take daily on an empty stomach. Alternatively use Artemisia (wormwood) oil, mixing with olive oil (or coconut oil) in the ratio of 1 8-10. Take at least 50 ml of this and repeat daily. One can also use Artemisia oil in an enema form, using 2ml of oil in about 100ml of lukewarm water. Another option when in the tropics is to use the sap of an unripe papaya.

See Chapter Nine: Homeopathic and Herbal Remedy list, Herbal and Plant remedies, Papaya section

A natural laxative should be taken at the same time, e.g., ripe fruit like figs, mangoes or papaya. Mix with lots of water and ideally take in the morning or empty stomach.

♦ HOMEOPATHIC CARE

Cina is the first remedy for irritable children with worms. There is great itching of the anus and violent boring and picking of the nose. Mentally the child is very angry and capricious. Nothing satisfies and the child is ugly and petulant, throwing things away when given. There can be grinding of teeth at night.

Sabadilla is good when there is great itching in the anus and skin and around the nose and ears. There is often itching in the palate of the mouth and twitching in many parts of the body. There is a watery, runny nose and eyes.

Teucrium marum verum is needed for itching of the anus, worse at night with crawling and picking of the nose. The child is over excitable and sensitive and has difficulty to sleep.

Silicea is for children who have worms with itching and who are losing weight with no appetite. They become more reserved and timid and avoid company due to a lack of confidence. They become more chilly and have profuse, sour perspiration.

Sulphur has great itching and burning in the anus and the skin in general, worse at night and when warm. There is offensive flatus and perspiration and the skin looks dirty. When no other remedy has relieved or only helped somewhat, *Sulphur* should be thought of.

NOTE Constitutional homeopathic care may be needed to fully resolve a worm infection. Sometimes homeopathic treatment is enough, either one of the remedies mentioned or a constitutional based remedy. However, conventional treatment can also be used.

Fasting or doing a prolonged juice fast can be a good way of helping purge worms from the system (but not to be done by children or those already malnourished due to chronic worm infection).

🍃 HERBAL CARE

There are a number of ways to purge parasites. One is to take two tbs. of black walnut hull tincture, seven capsules of wormwood (See Artemisia above) and one capsule of cloves three times a day. Parsley tea can also be used.

Essential Natural Health Guide

Chapter Six
Common Conditions

Allergies

Allergies are mostly due to a reaction of the body to external factors (pollen, trees, dust, animals, feathers, etc.), which creates a histamine reaction in the body, leading to a variety of symptoms mainly affecting the eyes, nose, throat, chest, and skin. Hayfever is an allergy that often occurs at particular times of the year. Contact dermatitis is an allergy to certain irritants exposed onto the skin. If an allergy looks like it is becoming serious and is affecting the respiration and or the throat, or it is known that a serious reaction can happen, for example, from a bee sting, immediate medical attention should be sought.

Food allergies are not discussed here in particular and normally require more constitutional treatment. However, in more acute situations, remedies can be given. *See Chapter Five, Digestive Conditions and Chapter Six, Eye Conditions.*

◆ HOMEOPATHIC CARE

Allergies can be treated two ways with homeopathy:

- Simply treating the acute symptoms while they are happening.
- Treating the underlying cause of the allergies, with 'constitutional' care. The focus here is on treating the acute symptoms.

Allium cepa is one of the main remedies for simple allergies. The focus is on the streaming eyes, which can burn and also profuse nasal discharge. There can be a tearing cough coming from the laryngeal area, feeling as if the throat is being torn apart.

Euphrasia and *Sabadilla* are two other similar remedies when the eyes and nose symptoms predominate. *Euphrasia* can also be taken in an eyedropper form. It has burning from the eyes and much streaming and often has inflammation of the conjunctiva of the eye.

Sabadilla treats similar eye and nose symptoms, but also profuse intense sneezing and there may be itching in the upper palate of the mouth.

Nux vomica is good when one feels extreme irritability with allergies and there is violent sneezing.

Arsenicum album is needed if there is much anxiety and restlessness, with burning of eyes, mouth, nose or skin.

Arum triphyllum is useful in hayfever and general allergies, when the nose is obstructed with acrid discharge and sneezing, with a great desire to pick and bore at the nose. There is great rawness in the mouth and throat and hawking from the throat and a hoarse voice.

Dulcamara is good for hayfever when symptoms are much worse after damp weather or when exposed to a damp climate or house, especially after having been heated and then suddenly chilled.

Apis, Urtica urens and *Rhus tox* are indicated if allergies are on the skin. *Apis* is the first remedy to think of for a serious systemic allergy when the respiration is affected and threatens to close up the throat. There may be intense, burning, stinging and puffiness on the skin, especially around the eyes and there can be heat and a craving for open air. This is the remedy for threatened anaphylaxis when you may need immediate medical intervention. Give *Apis* in a 200c potency ideally, in water every one minute and get medical attention.

Urtica urens is a good remedy for food allergies with hives which burn and itch. A shellfish allergy in particular indicates this remedy.

Rhus tox is good for skin symptoms with many blisters (vesicles) and for intense burning, itching and restlessness
Remedies can be taken one to five times a day depending on severity of symptoms. If more than twice a day, take the remedy in water and take one tsp. for each dose.
See Chapter Seven: Skin Conditions, Poison oak.

COMBINATION STRATEGY If you cannot find one remedy to match the symptoms you are feeling, then put one tablet of each indicated remedy into two to four ounces of water and take one sip three to five times daily for two to three days or until relief.

Breast and Vaginal Issues

This may include inflammation of the breast (mastitis) due to breast feeding problems, or other breast feeding issues. For breast abscesses, also refer to *Chapter Seven: Skin Conditions, Boils section*. For injuries to the breast, also look at *Chapter Three: Accidents, Injuries and Trauma*. If lumps remain after a significant blow to the breast or there is bleeding from the nipple for any reason, seek medical advice.

For acute vaginal herpetic eruptions or candida, a topical use of neem oil mixed with yoghurt and olive oil can help. Also Wild oregano oil can be used topically (diluted with a neutral oil) and also taken internally. Homeopathic remedies such as ***Rhus tox*** or ***Dulcamara*** can be given for an acute herpetic eruption, but constitutional care is ideally needed.

◆ HOMEOPATHIC CARE

Belladonna is the remedy for acute inflammation of the breast, when there is great heat, redness and burning, and the pain is worse from any motion.

Bryonia is needed if there is hardness in the breast, along with heat, but not as intense as **Belladonna** and where any motion makes it worse. **Phytolacca** is needed if the breast is extremely hard, perhaps with nodules and pain and swelling extends into the armpit and the nipples may be cracked, .

Phytolacca is also the first remedy to give where there is any hardness of the breast and in simple blocked ducts when breast feeding, It is also the first remedy for abscesses in the breasts that are complications of mastitis and/or blocked ducts. There can be painful cracks in the nipples as mentioned.

Urtica urens is needed when milk decreases or stops in one breast, with no other symptoms.

Pulsatilla is needed if there is much weepiness and emotion along with problems with breast feeding. There may be not enough milk or after weaning the child, the milk continues. There may be an increased desire to walk in the open air, or simply for fresh air.

Silicea may be needed (for the mother) if the baby refuses to take the milk or vomits after feeding. It seems the milk is not good for the child. There can be sharp pains in the breasts and inflammation and hardness of the breast.

Bellis perennis can be used for any injury to the breast, especially when involving a blow which leaves a lump, . It is similar to **Arnica** and from the same botanical family. Use **Arnica** if you don't have **Bellis perennis**. Another remedy for residual lumps in the breast from blows is **Conium** but it is best to get professional homeopathic advice. For thrush on the nipples of nursing women when the baby also has thrush, take **Borax**.

HERBAL CARE

Vervaine (*Verbena officianalis*) can be given in tea form to help stimulate milk production, especially when feeling exhausted from too much stress and care. Nettle tea (*Urtica urens*) can also be given in tea form to do the same thing. Nettle is an amazing herb and is full of vitamins and minerals. Asafœtida tea promotes production of breast milk.

Colds

A cold is the generic term given for an infection, usually viral, which affects the eyes, nose and throat. It can lead to secondary infections of the sinuses, larynx/trachea and lungs. When traveling, 'new' viruses tend to afflict people with unusual colds. There may be a general fever but also it can be localized in the head region with no fever. If there is a cough with the cold, look at the Cough section for more remedy descriptions.

GENERAL CARE

Rest as much as possible. Do not take long trips or expose yourself to the cold and general elements. Drink plenty of fluids, both cold and hot, and eat well. If the nose is very congested, use steam to help open up the breathing passageways.

HOMEOPATHIC CARE

It is good to pay attention to the type of weather if you catch a cold as it can help in finding a remedy.

Aconite is the most likely remedy in cold, dry weather or when exposed to a cold wind and symptoms come on suddenly, with perhaps a fever, heat and chill. There may be all the normal symptoms of a runny nose etc., but the key symptoms are the suddenness of the symptoms, with a burning fever, intense thirst and mentally restless and anxious.

Arsenicum album can look very similar but often the discharge from the eyes and nose is more burning and acrid, the symptoms don't come on so quickly and intensely but there is chilliness and restlessness, often being more chilly than *Aconite*. The key is the focus on the eyes and nose, along with chilliness and restlessness.

Nux vomica also looks like *Arsenicum album*, but has more intense sneezing and less burning of the eyes and nose. There can be great irritability with symptoms and feelings of great chill with shaking, which becomes worse when drinking cold drinks.

Allium cepa is the classic remedy for a cold when all the symptoms revolve around the eyes, nose and throat, with great watering of the eyes and nose and great irritation and burning in the eyes. There can be a tickling cough coming from the larynx, with a tearing pain when coughing, which is often worse in a warm room.

Sabadilla is very similar to *Allium cepa*, but has more violent sneezing and also itching of the upper mouth (palate).

🌿 HERBAL CARE

Take *echinacea* and/or goldenseal tincture ten drops hourly for one day. Also take ginger tea. Take the echinacea for up to ten days. It is most effective when taken at the beginning of a cold. Eucalyptus oil can be used as an inhaler, with some drops put into hot water and steamed.

Coughs
including bronchitis and pneumonia

Coughs occur for many reasons and it is important to know the reasons for the cough, whether it is just a mild, self-limiting condition or indicative of something more serious, e.g., pneumonia. Often, it is associated with some of kind of bacterial or viral infection. The following are the most obvious remedies for many coughs, including whooping cough. If whooping cough is seen in a small child, it is important to have professional medical care available. It is useful to look at the cold, fever and influenza sections for more remedies as coughs are often part of a cold and/ or influenza. It is not always easy to find the right homeopathic remedy for a cough. It is very important to find out what features make the cough worse or better, e.g., warm or cold weather, food or drink, talking, lying down, sitting up, etc. Also, pay attention to what the cough sounds and feels like, e.g., hacking, dry, wet, racking, barking etc. All this helps in choosing the correct remedy. You are becoming a homeopath!

Bronchitis is a bacterial infection in the bronchioles of the lung, leading at times to a fever, intense cough, exhaustion and general depletion. It may occur after a more superficial cold has gone 'deeper' into the lungs. It can become a chronic condition or can frequently recur in people sensitive to the condition. Often it is experienced as an intense cough that does not seem to go away by itself. It may or may not be associated with a fever. Remedies suggested include those for pneumonia, a deeper infection of the lungs than bronchitis. This can require medical intervention, especially in elderly people and when as a complication of influenza or other general infections.

● **GENERAL CARE**

Ensure enough water is taken for hydration. Keep warm. Do not move too much or aggravate the cough by violent exertion. Try and allow the mucus to come up, if there is some. Warm drinks may help loosen mucus. Use lozenges if necessary. If the cough is dry and irritating and especially worse at night, mix some honey, cider vinegar and a pinch of cayenne pepper together in a small amount of hot water and sip as needed. Other natural methods may work as well.

It is very distressing when children experience a sudden, intense cough. Croup (a cough with a spasm in the larynx causing breathing to be impeded) can be very intense as it seems the child is suffocating. Then suddenly the child will breathe in deeply making a strange sound and is then relieved from bit. It is important to sit the child up. Attacks happen mostly at night and in children older than two years. The cough itself is hard, barking, violent and the cough seems to be suffocating the child. It is important to know if this is just a case of croup or whether the suffocative breathing is due to any other factor, including something stuck in the air passage. Whooping cough is also very similar to this and the same remedies are indicated although whooping cough is most serious in infants. There is also a condition where the epiglottis is swollen at the back of the tongue and this may be interfering with breathing. Immediate medical care should be sought. *Aconite* should be given to help matters while waiting for medical care.

● HOMEOPATHIC CARE

The most important factors in choosing which remedy you need are the sound of the cough and what makes it better or worse. This is the same whether we are looking at whooping cough, croup, bronchitis, pneumonia or just a simple cough. However, knowing the type and depth of infection can be important in helping identifying the remedy and also when a more serious infection is taking place. *Aconite*, *Drosera* and *Hepar sulph* are important remedies when there is a cough that is hard, barking, choking, or like a croup. In *Aconite*, the cough may come on very quickly and is often worse at night. Any cough with intense fear and anxiety indicates *Aconite*.

Drosera is one of the best remedies for many types of cough, especially when it is barking and hard. It is the first remedy to think of for whooping cough. There can even be retching and vomiting with the cough and it is often worse at night as soon as the head hits the pillow. *Cuprum metallicum* and *Ipecac* are two other important remedies in whooping cough. In both remedies the face can turn red or blue on coughing and in *Cuprum* the cough comes in violent spasms and with cramps in the body and may be better from cold drinks. Both can have loud rattling in the chest. See below for *Ipecac*.

Hepar sulph has a similar sounding cough but it is much worse from any cold air and better from warm drinks. One may even hear a rattle in the chest with great choking.

Spongia is another remedy that has a very characteristic barking cough, which is like a seal bark or a saw going through wood. It is excellent for whooping cough and croup and when there is great dryness in the larynx/trachea area. The cough is better from drinking cold water.

Bryonia has one of the most painful of coughs and either the head, throat and chest needs to be held while coughing, similar to *Drosera* and *Phosphorus*. The cough of *Drosera* can sound similar. Any movement makes it worse and the cough is mostly dry, hard and hacking and is often worse in a warm room.

Belladonna is similar to *Bryonia* with a dry, intense, painful and barking cough and both can have fever with the cough. They are important remedies in the first stages of bronchitis, especially when fever comes with the cough. There can be a great desire to drink due to dryness in the mouth and throat.

Arsenicum album is indicated when along with the cough there is a great burning feeling in the chest and also much restlessness and anxiety. Burning may also be felt in all the mucus membranes and the cough is mostly dry and hacking and often worse around midnight.

Phosphorus has a cough that is usually dry and hacking and often there is tightness and a feeling of emptiness in the chest. The cough is often worse from a change in temperature, going from warm to cold or vice versa. It is one of the most important remedies in bronchitis and pneumonia and when intense the cough can rack the whole body. The person suffering often feels weak and exhausted.

Ipecac and *Pulsatilla* have a much looser, more rattling type of cough. In *Ipecac*, the rattling cough often comes with nausea, retching and vomiting, the face turning red when coughing. There can be a sense of suffocating with the cough and it is needed in croup, whooping cough, bronchitis and pneumonia. It can be hard to bring mucus up, even with rattling. In croup and whooping cough it is similar to *Drosera*. *Coccus cacti* is also similar, with production of much stringy, sticky mucus with the cough and/ or has intense vomiting along with the mucus. The cough is intensely tickling and violent, with a red face with the cough.

Pulsatilla has a cough that is often associated with other conditions, such as conjunctivitis, sinusitis, otitis media or bronchitis. It is mostly loose and mucus from the chest or nose is yellow and/or yellow/green. It is much worse in a warm room and better in the open air and is also much worse from lying down. *Pulsatilla* is a great children's remedy for coughs and colds and fever especially coming after getting wet feet.

If bronchitis has moved to becoming pneumonia and there is great exhaustion and inability to recover, then a few other remedies are useful.

Antimonium tart is excellent for pneumonia when one feels as if drowning in mucus and can't get enough breath. The cough is deep, loose and suffocating, along with great rattling and wheezing. It is very hard to bring up mucus and it is exhausting trying to do so, making one pale and sweaty. It feels as if one's lungs are becoming paralyzed.

Carbo vegetabilis is another remedy when one is really struggling with the cough. There is total exhaustion, sweat and coldness and as if one can't get enough oxygen. There is a desire to be fanned, even though cold. The face may turn blue but feel burning and rattling in the lungs.

Lachesis is a similar state, with blueness of the face and where there is blood in the sputum being coughed up. The breathing is characteristically much worse on falling asleep and on waking.

If some of these remedies have been given and only worked partially and it is hard to get back to normal, then you should give *Sulphur* three times a day for three days. There may be residual burning in the lungs, weakness and the cough often wakes you at night.

COMBINATION STRATEGY If you are unsure of which remedy and the cough is croupy, choking and/or barking in nature, combine one tablet of *Aconite*, *Drosera* and *Hepar sulph* in water and take two to four times a day, depending on the intensity of the cough. If that doesn't work give *Spongia*. If it is pneumonia, with great weakness and a loose, rattling cough, which makes the person feel as if suffocating, you can combine *Antimonium tart*, *Carbo veg* and *Ipecac* and take as described above. In whooping cough, one can add *Drosera, Cuprum* and *Ipecac* together if not sure.

🌿 HERBAL CARE

Eucalyptus oil can be inhaled with bronchitis and with general colds. Do not inhale at the same time as taking a homeopathic remedy.

Cystitis

Cystitis is an infection of the bladder, due to a bacterial infection. It may be caused by having sex, by being unable to wash frequently, by heat, or it can be due to a more chronic vulnerability. In the latter case, constitutional homeopathic care is needed. It is important to see if there is any pain in the mid back region, which could indicate the infection going to the kidney. *See Kidney section.* If that is the case, seek medical attention. At times, the infection can begin in the kidney. In an acute kidney infection, one should see relief from fever and pain in about two to three hours. If there is no change in four hours, in any way, choose another remedy. If there is some change, even if slight, continue with the remedy. In cystitis, improvement may take longer but some change should be seen between four hours and one day, depending on the severity of the symptoms.

● GENERAL CARE

At the first sign of symptoms, drink a lot of water. Cranberry juice is often used as well and seems to help avert the condition. Avoid alcohol and acidic drinks. Symptoms are usually a combination of an increased urging to urinate, burning pain in the urethra before, during and/or after urination, occasional fever, general sick feeling, aching in the bladder and back pain. The urine may be cloudy, bloody, with an offensive odor. The urging to urinate may be very intense, but with little urine being passed.

If you develop blood in the urine or begin to suffer from cystitis, kidney stones, prostate or uterine infections and have spent time in Africa and other tropical regions within two years, then bilharzia should be considered.

See Chapter Eight: Tropical Conditions, Bilharzia.

● HOMEOPATHIC CARE

Staphysagria is needed for simple cystitis that comes from having sex.

Cantharis is needed when very intense symptoms begin very quickly, with a violent, constant urging, but only a few drops are passed, or the urine is bloody. It is also needed if the infection goes into the kidneys.

Berberis is needed when there are pains in the kidneys along with the cystitis with pains radiating outwards from the bladder region and often extending down the legs and to the kidneys. Pains are always changing place. *Berberis* is needed when the kidney is the primary area affected with burning pains and pains radiating down toward the bladder and into the back. It is one of the first remedies for kidney stones with intense colicky pains.

Lycopodium is a good kidney colic remedy, when the right side is affected and there is red sand in the urine. There may be abdominal symptoms seen, which is described in *Chapter Five: Digestive Conditions, Hepatitis section.*

Equisetum is a good for cystitis when the strongest symptom is simply a great fullness in the bladder which is not relieved when urinating.

Nux vomica is needed when there is an intense, cutting, violent, stitching pain in the kidney region, and a strong urging to urinate but little passes. It is also a kidney colic remedy. It sounds similar to *Cantharis*, but the symptoms indicating *Cantharis* are even more intense and frenzied and there is more blood in the urine. *See Chapter Five, Digestive conditions.*

Sarsaparilla is useful when none of the other remedies seem indicated or haven't worked. It is one of the most indicated remedies in cystitis. Often, the burning pain is felt right at the end of urination and there can be a chill feeling spreading up the urethra to the bladder. One may have the strange experience of feeling gas pass from the bladder.

Apis is an important remedy for acute kidney infection (nephritis), especially when it comes on suddenly, with great burning, stinging and a fever but with no thirst. One may see a strange puffiness around the eyelids. There can a bursting feeling in the bladder and kidney, with fullness of the bladder and hot urine.

Belladonna is needed when cystitis comes on very quickly and intensely, with burning and a hot, dry fever. Pains are often throbbing and the urine is also burning.

COMBINATION STRATEGY If in doubt as to which remedy to give, put one tablet of each remedy that seems indicated into a glass of water, and sip the glass frequently (every fifteen to thirty minutes depending on the severity of symptoms). Stir the water before taking each sip. For a kidney infection, if no remedy is clear, use **Apis**, **Berberis**, **Cantharis** and **Nux vomica** together. Put one tablet of each remedy in a glass of water and take a sip every ten minutes until some relief is felt, stirring the water each time. Change should be noticed in one to two hours.

✐ HERBAL CARE

Take one or more of the following, either in a tea or tincture: Uva ursi, dandelion leaf, marshmallow root, juniper root or horsetail. Goldenrod is also very useful. Cranberry can be taken, either in juice form or tablets. It is useful to prevent a urinary infection get any worse.

Ear Pain

Ear pain is often a result of an accumulation of mucus behind the ear drum, creating pressure and pain. There may a bacterial infection involved or it may be a consequence of a general viral infection which may lead to a secondary bacterial infection. An inner ear infection is called otitis media. Antibiotics are commonly given, especially for children, but often there is no bacterial infection so they do not work in those cases. Pain may also be caused by inflammation in the outer canal of the ear that leads to the eardrum. This is more easily treatable and less serious than an inner ear infection and is due to bacterial or fungal infection, often because of a tropical climate and hygiene challenges.

● GENERAL CARE

If there is a general fever, do not routinely give anti-inflammatory medicines, (tylenol etc.). A fever is a natural reaction of the body. It should only be suppressed if the fever is very high, or the person (especially a child) is in severe discomfort. It is hard to watch a child suffer so using homeopathic remedies along with anti-inflammatory medicines is OK. Treat the fever by keeping the person cool, using a cool wash cloth and even taking a tepid bath. Keep the person hydrated. Drinking water is extremely important. When lying down, lie on the opposite side to the ear pain. For external ear infections clean well, using *Calendula* or *Hypericum* tincture in warm water. Be careful not to push anything too far into the ear such as cotton plugs etc.

● HOMEOPATHIC CARE

There are many remedies for acute ear pain/infection. *Aconite* and *Belladonna* are often needed when there is a sudden attack of ear pain, the pain comes suddenly and is often associated with a fever. *Aconite* is the first remedy when symptoms come on after exposure to a cold wind and then suddenly there is great pain in the ear and a high fever.

Belladonna is good for a bursting, throbbing pain in the ear and the fever is mostly dry, burning and with a red face or ear.

Hepar sulph and *Mercurius* are needed when there is an infection with the accumulation of pus behind the ear. The fever is not so high as *Aconite* or *Belladonna*, but both remedies have a sharp, stitching pain in the ear and the pain is worse from swallowing.

Hepar sulph has pain like a splinter in the ear. The pain often moves from the ear to the throat and back and the pain is much worse from any swallowing and one feels very chilly in general. The ear pain is better from warm applications and worse from any cold. One can feel very touchy and angry and there can be offensive discharge from the ear.

Mercurius is one of the great ear, nose and throat remedies and often ear problems are connected to throat infections. There is often offensive breath and a metallic taste, with increased salivation, especially at night. There can be a low fever, often alternating with a chill, with shaking and trembling and offensive perspiration. *Mercurius* can often be given after *Hepar sulph* if it has not finished the job.

Chamomilla and *Pulsatilla* are two other remedies to consider. *Chamomilla* is known as a remedy for all sorts of pain. When one needs *Chamomilla*, one can feel the pain is unendurable. Nothing seems to relieve it. It is one of the first remedies to give to children with ear pains. Mentally, the child can be angry, capricious and does not want to be touched or disturbed. The child often shrieks with the pain. The same applies if seen in an adult.

Pulsatilla has a different mental state. The child feels weepy, helpless, whiny and demanding. There can often be yellow/green discharge from the ear or nose and it may start after having wet and cold feet. The pain is often worse in a warm room and is better in the open air.

Sulphur should be considered when other remedies have not totally worked or you simply don't feel yourself. There is a lack of energy and interest. There may be some burning and pressure in the ear.

COMBINATION STRATEGY If the symptoms are intense, acute, and there is a general fever, you can combine *Aconite*, *Chamomilla* and *Belladonna*, one tablet of each in two to four ounces of water, one tsp. taken every fifteen to sixty minutes until relief sets in. Follow with *Sulphur* if this does not work. *Hepar sulph* and *Mercurius* can also be mixed if you cannot make a distinction.

✐ HERBAL CARE

Use garlic/mullein ear oil, putting into the ear following instructions on the bottle. Plantago tincture may also be used.

Ear Injury

One should be very careful when dealing with any injury in the ear. Do not poke or put anything into the ear. One can easily injure the ear drum, even leading to perforation. If a drum is perforated, then also putting anything into the ear can lead to infection. If a foreign object is in the ear get professional attention. If this is not available, apply a gentle syringing of warm water with *Calendula* tincture added. Do not syringe directly into the center of the ear, but toward the top and let the liquid go down into the ear. If there is an abrasion to parts of the canal leading to the eardrum, wash carefully with warm water and *Calendula* and use *Calendula* cream after. Be very careful if putting *Calendula* on with a Q tip. If there is excessive wax in the ear, you can use a little mullein oil warmed on a hot spoon and gently put into the ear over a number of days to loosen the wax. For any pain in the ear, or anxiety consider giving *Aconite* or *Chamomilla*.

Eye Conditions

Blepharitis

Blepharitis in an infection of the margins of the eyelids. Although it can be an acute condition, it often recurs in a more chronic condition and requires constitutional homeopathic care to treat effectively.

Conjunctivitis

Conjunctivitis is often a bacterial infection in the conjunctiva (the lining) of the eye, although viral forms exist. It may be the consequence of allergies and other irritations to the eye. Children often get this condition, called 'pinkeye'. It is mostly treated with topical antibiotics. It tends to be highly infectious.

Styes and Chalazae

A stye is an inflamed lump/tumor found near the edge of the eyelid caused by a bacterial infection, often in the root of an eyelash. It can arise as an acute condition but often has a recurring chronic tendency. Symptoms are mainly an inflammation of the upper and/or lower eyelid, with swelling redness and itching. There are often hard nodules on the eyelid. A chalazion is a lump on the eyelid due to a blocked oil gland. It is normally larger than a stye, it doesn't hurt but can impede vision if large. It will normally go away of itself in time. A stye tends to be more toward the edge of the eyelid.

● GENERAL CARE

With conjunctivitis wash the eye well with warm water. Avoid contagion by washing hands frequently. Use homeopathic or other natural eye drops with *Euphrasia* (eyebright) in to help with the infection. With styes and chalazion, use warm compresses a few times a day. This may help open the pores, relieving the symptoms. Don't squeeze the stye or chalazion to try and open it. For babies with conjunctivitis, use breast milk.

◆ HOMEOPATHIC CARE

Euphrasia. is the first remedy for simple conjunctivitis. Symptoms are burning and swelling of eyes and eyelids. There may be yellow and/or watery discharge from the eyes.

Pulsatilla is also indicated for thick yellow/green discharge from the eyes. This is useful for children who are weepy, mild and clingy when sick. It is also a good remedy for simple styes, especially if found near the inner corner of the eyes. If there is a blocked tear duct, which is not uncommon in new born babies, leading to yellowy/green discharge from the eye, you can try *Pulsatilla* or *Silicea* if that doesn't work. If it persists, you should seek professional care.

Allium cepa can be given when there is excessive watering of the eyes and burning pain, but the discharge is bland. There can be great sensitivity to the light.

Belladonna can be used when the eyes are very red, congested, with burning, fullness and great heat. The pupils are dilated.

Staphysagria is given more for blepharitis occurring with styes or chalazae. The styes are hard and there are nodules on the lids which are itching. If a stye comes after an emotional upset or quarrel, then this is a good remedy.

Sulphur is given when there is burning and dryness in the eye and it feels inflamed and swollen and may itch a lot, especially in a warm room.

🍃 HERBAL CARE

Using an eye tincture of *Euphrasia* (eyebright) and/or *Hamamelis* (witch-hazel) is very good.

Eye Injury

♦ HOMEOPATHIC CARE

Arnica is the first remedy to give for a simple black eye, due to injury. If that doesn't clear everything up and bruising and swelling remain, you should give *Ledum*. *Ledum* is also useful for any injury due to a pointed object in the eye.

Symphytum is useful for injury to the bone around the eye. It also follows *Arnica* well. Any serious injury to the eye and the face, including the bones of the face and skull should be checked as soon as possible by a medical expert. There may be a skull fracture.

If there is any foreign body in the eye, the eye can be bathed in an eyebath using three drops of either *Calendula*, *Hamamelis* or *Hypericum* tincture. For any pain or inflammation in the eye, from an object, injury or otherwise, *Euphrasia* (or similar eye mixture that has *Euphrasia* as one of the ingredients) should be used as an eyebath. *Euphrasia* in a 6c or 30c homeopathic potency can be used at the same time.

Ruta grav is indicated for simple eyestrain due to overexertion of using the eyes, perhaps reading in the dark or doing really fine work, then use, three times a day for three days.

Simple Fever

Any common infection that involves a fever can be found here and influenza is also included in this chapter and needs to be studied along with the fever remedies. There are many reasons for fevers to occur, influenza being one of the most common, so identifying the key characteristics of remedies for both conditions is useful to know. In homeopathy a remedy is given based on the unique symptom picture, not the name of the disease.

A fever is a natural body reaction to any type of infection. It is the way the body 'throws off' a disease through an increased level of activity of the body's immune system. It is important to find out why the fever is there. Which area is affected? Is there pain associated with the fever? It is good not to simply suppress a fever. There is a tendency to always want to do something. It is better to try and let the fever take its course or give the correct homeopathic remedy if the picture is clear.

Fevers are most often seen in children. Fevers up to 104f, (40 Celsius) are not unusual and if it comes down to around 100f (37.5 Celsius) fairly quickly after treatment, there is normally nothing to worry about. Fevers higher than 104f or which don't come down after treatment may require professional care. Any sign of a stiff neck, arching of the neck or pain in the area requires medical intervention as it may be meningitis.

Fevers occur in adults most often when having the 'flu, stomach conditions or when traveling due to a more serious tropical disease. Although the temperature may go as high as 104f (40 C), it is usually less than this. In most cases, do not suppress the fever with drugs. Take appropriate care and treatment and wait it out. Exceptions are when fever is associated with a potentially serious condition such as a kidney infection, blood poisoning, malaria or other serious infection in a part of the body. In these cases, there should be other symptoms to indicate the nature of the problem.

● GENERAL CARE

Explore the possible causes of the fever – is there pain anywhere, swelling, or any other symptom? With viral cold infections, fever is often a generalized response to the virus and there is no specific area affected. With a fever, keep hydrated. Drink plenty of water. Take rehydration salts if any fever lasts more than 12 hours or is extremely intense. Do not get exposed to the cold. Keep warm, especially if the fever involves a chill. Eat only small amounts, if at all. If necessary, take a tepid bath or do a sponge bath with tepid water if the fever is exceptionally high. Cool the head down if there is heat. Do not let children get too hot with a fever but also refrain from using too many medications to suppress a fever unless it is very high. However, if the fever does not go down in a number of days or is getting exceptionally high, seek professional medical care.

● HOMEOPATHIC CARE

Many other remedies can have fever associated with them, but are not listed here. The remedies listed here are known for their fever symptoms alone, whereas with other remedies there will be other information to prescribe on. See the listed chapters above and also the Influenza section. It is important to check the area that may be infected, e.g., ear, bladder, throat etc., as there are other remedies that will be listed there which are more specific for those conditions. The remedies listed below are the main ones for a simple fever.

Aconite and *Belladonna* are often needed if the fever comes on very suddenly and intensely. *Aconite* has a high, often dry fever, with great thirst and much restlessness, anxiety and even anguish. Exposure to cold air may often be the cause of an *Aconite* type fever. There may an intense inflammatory process or disease, e.g., acute ear infection and much pain can be seen. Everything feels extreme and if it comes after an intense emotional shock, this confirms the remedy.

Belladonna has a classic intense hot fever. One can feel as if burning up inside, the skin is hot and dry, the face flushed, the eyes staring and the pupils are dilated. It is often needed in children who suddenly spike a fever. There can be thirst for small sips or large amounts and even for lemonade. There can even be wild delirium with thrashing about and this is worse from any motion and jarring. It is the first remedy to consider for any sudden fever.

Apis can also be given for fevers. Often it looks like *Belladonna* and there is often no thirst, even though very hot or the thirst comes when feeling chilled. If *Apis* is needed, it may indicate an infection of some other organ, e.g., kidney or bladder. Pains may be burning and stinging, and in the fever, the head is rolling from side to side. The skin will often be dark or bright red.

Bryonia, *Eupatorium perfoliatum* and *Gelsemium* have fevers that do not come on so suddenly or intensely. They develop more slowly but can also get quite high. In *Bryonia*, there is great dryness of the body and the mucous membranes, leading to a large thirst. There can also be delirium, at times saying "I want to go home", when already there. They often want to keep totally still, are worse from any jar and can be irritable and want to be left alone.

Eupatorium and *Gelsemium* are similar in that they both have extreme aching of the muscles and joints with the fever. That is why they are good 'flu remedies. Both remedies can have a strong chill, which goes up and down the back. *Eupatorium* often has more thirst than *Gelsemium* which can be thirstless. The pains in *Eupatorium* feel like their bones are breaking, most often felt in the back. There can also be nausea and vomiting with the fever, even of bile. Nausea is worse from the smell of food.

Gelsemium has the intense aching of muscles and often feels sleepy, weak, dizzy and dull. The face can be besotted (confused and full looking), looking very dull and the eyelids feel too heavy to hold up, and even the head can feel too heavy to hold up.

Nux vomica is a great remedy for any fever associated with a 'stomach 'flu'. With the fever, there is great chill, wanting to be covered at all times and worse from any drafts, which is similar to *Arsenicum album* and *Rhus tox*. *See Influenza below.* There can be much cramping in the stomach or back area and very irritable and sensitive to any noise and smells. All senses are more acute.

Sulphur is needed when there is burning and throbbing of any part of the body with the fever and an indifference and disconnection to what is going on around one. It is good when there doesn't seem a clear picture for any other remedy but something is definitely going on.

🍃 HERBAL CARE

Make a tea with a combination of elderflower, yarrow and peppermint. Also boneset tea can be used. Using eucalyptus and tea tree oil in fevers and 'flu can be useful, adding it to some steaming water for a vapor effect. Elderberry juice has been used for generations against fever, influenza and other viral and bacterial conditions. Lemon grass tea is good to take for any fever, one to two liters per day.

Influenza

We often say we have the 'flu when we simply have a bad cold. True influenza is due to particular viruses and historically we have been getting forms of the 'flu for thousands of years. Spread from animals such as birds and pigs, they have contaminated humans and led to outbreaks of influenza.

There are various strains of influenza, creating the challenge to find a vaccine for the current strain, which changes each year. They are classified according to their make-up, and given titles such as H1N1, H5N1 etc. This relates to the genetic code of the virus. However, whatever type of 'flu it is, they are relatively mild for most people and can be treated effectively with homeopathy. A healthy constitution generally helps mitigate more serious complications of most 'flus. The most serious and frequent complication of the 'flu is pneumonia, which occurs mainly in children under two and in seniors. The viral form of pneumonia can be very serious and requires instant treatment. It comes on very quickly whereas bacterial pneumonia is slower to develop.

The fear today is of a new strain of 'flu virus arriving that we have no genetic immunity to, contaminating humans through connections with certain animals and then mutating into a virulent form of the virus, similar to the 1918 'Spanish 'flu' epidemic, in which up to 30 million people died. In the normal course of affairs, once someone has had the 'flu, immunity is developed to the same strain and even to slightly different strains. The concern is when a totally different strain is seen which would affect healthy young people as much as the elderly and infants.

The effectiveness of influenza vaccines being offered varies from year to year and the overall effectiveness is disputable. In the elderly, the original focus for the vaccine, the lack of effectiveness can be due to their diminishing immune response due to age. According to the Centers for Disease Control (CDC), the effectiveness of the 'flu vaccine among elderly in nursing homes is 30-40%. It may be even lower than that. Also, the 'flu vaccines do have significant side effects, which are often not admitted by the medical profession, dimishing the acttual facts of the vaccine's effect. Inspite of the growing pressure to get flu vaccines, healthy people should not be overly concerned.

Due to the increased concern of a new virulent form of influenza, one should ensure all precautions are taken against the 'flu and also to treat any symptoms effectively. Anti viral treatments may work against some 'flu viruses but there are no guarantees. The effect of Tamiflu, for example, is already very limited in many cases.

● GENERAL CARE

It is important to rest when signs of the 'flu are there and to keep hydrated. Do not get overexposed to the cold and keep warm.

◆ HOMEOPATHIC CARE

The remedies mentioned are similar for many other types of viral and bacterial infections. The most important thing is to identify the main characteristics of each remedy, irrespective of the name of the condition. Remedies have been separated according to certain stages of the 'flu which are often seen. *See Colds and Coughs.*

1st stage of symptoms when high fever predominates.

All remedies in the *Fever section* can be considered here. However, in the first stages when symptoms develop, if it is an intense and sudden onset of symptoms with fever, then *Aconite* and *Belladonna* are the most common remedies. The intensity of heat, high fever, thirst and throbbing congestion of blood, especially in the head are important symptoms. *Aconite* is more restless, anxious and fearful and the thirst is stronger. In *Belladonna* there can be more wildness and delirium with the fever, often with dilated pupils, a red complexion and a wild look in the face.

Bryonia also has heat and a bad headache, like *Belladonna* but the symptoms develop more slowly and they are more irritable, desire to be left alone and also like *Belladonna* don't want to be moved at all. They can have delirium as well, but it is more passive.

Arsenicum album has fever and heat alternating with chill and extreme restlessness and anxiety.

Rhus tox also has great restlessness and also heat alternating with chill. The chill is worse for any uncovering and the restlessness is less to do with anxiety and more simply a need to move around. Both *Arsenicum* and *Rhus tox* can be restless during fever and especially at night in bed. *Rhus tox* also has a strange symptom of redness on the tip of the tongue, while *Arsenicum album* may have a white coated tongue, like paint.

1st stage with fever but body aching predominates. (Also include remedies above)

Gelsemium is the most commonly prescribed remedy for 'flu when aching of the body predominates. The aching is felt in the muscles all over the body, but especially the back. There is fever and chills, which are felt especially going up and down the back. Often with fever, there is no thirst. The strongest symptoms are aching, with drowsiness, dullness and a weak feeling. Even the eyelids seem too heavy to hold open.

Eupatorium perfoliatum can often look like *Gelsemium*. However the aching is felt more in the bones, as if they are breaking. It is a deep ache and often felt in the back. There is also fever and chill, and like *Gelsemium*, it goes up and down the back. There can be intense shaking with the chill and also nausea and vomiting, even of bile. *Bryonia* and *Rhus tox* can also have intense aching and are described above.

Arnica and *Baptisia* can be given when there is great soreness and a bruised feeling with aching, great exhaustion and an ongoing state of low fever in protracted 'flu. In *Arnica* one feels sore and averse to be touched or even approached. The bed can feel too hard with much tossing and turning. That feeling of the bed being too hard is common to both remedies.

Baptisia has great weakness, drowsiness and feeling extremely languid. It is like *Gelsemium* but even more weak and prostrated. In a fever state, one can feel as if parts of the body are scattered about the bed. There can be a foul odor of the body and a septic feeling in the body. There may be diarrhea/dysentery with 'flu symptoms. These remedies are also indicated in tropical diseases such as typhoid. *See Chapter Nine Tropical Diseases.*

2nd stage when weakness, exhaustion and depletion predominate.

For symptom pictures, see above. This weak state may come on quickly in a 'flu state or may develop more slowly as the condition gets worse and you feel as if you are sinking deeper into the condition.

Arsenicum album and *Rhus tox* can be thought of if the weakness come on quickly. *Gelsemium* is often the remedy if symptoms develop more slowly.

Arnica, *Baptisia* and also *Pyrogen* can be thought of however in more serious states with great weakness and prostration, This last remedy looks like *Baptisia*, has great soreness and also low fever with offensive discharges and odor. It feels septic and is useful for any fever that comes from a septic infection. One symptom is that the pulse can either be much too quick or too slow for the condition. It is often indicated in serious conditions like typhoid, malaria or pelvic infections.

3rd stage when lung symptoms predominate, including hemorrhage and pneumonia

This is a very serious stage of the 'flu and can be caused by other infections. Appropriate medical care should be sought. Homeopathy can be used alongside conventional treatment. Check for remedy information in *Colds, Coughs and Fever sections*.

COMBINATION STRATEGY You can combine one or more remedies that seem similar to the symptoms being seen. It is not always easy to find the exact remedy but look for the most important characteristics to help make a decision. Mix one tablet of the remedies chosen into a glass of water, and take one tsp. every one to four hours, depending on the severity of symptoms. Some change should be seen between 12-24 hours but it may take a couple of days to feel real improvement.

NOTE Professional homeopathic and other medical care should be sought to address serious conditions and also for any consequences after the 'flu. Some people find it very difficult to recover after serious 'flu and their immune systems remain low for a period of time. Homeopathy can be effective in addressing this situation.

✐ HERBAL CARE

Echinacea tincture 30 drops hourly or three to four times a day depending on severity of symptoms. It can also be taken to prevent the 'flu and can be taken in a homeopathic dose for ailments that have stemmed from the 'flu. As mentioned for fever, eucalyptus and tea tree oil can be used in hot water. Elderberry juice can be taken as well. Ginger and cinnamon tea can be taken.

Taking larger doses of Vitamin C are often taken to help prevent and address 'flu symptoms. Vitamin D3 can be taken during the 'flu season as prevention.

Kidney Disease

Inflammation of the kidneys is a potentially serious condition and requires immediate medical treatment if possible. It can stem from a bladder infection which then moves to the kidney or may be due to a blockage in one of the ureters (the tubes coming from the kidney and going to the bladder). Stones coming from the kidney can get stuck in the ureter leading to excruciating pain. Kidney infections may be due to some underlying vulnerability in the region. Kidney stones tend to begin with sudden, intense pain, and without fever or burning urination. A kidney stone may require surgical intervention and needs to be medically diagnosed.

● GENERAL CARE

Especially in kidney stones, one should drink a lot of fluid. Ideally this will help pass the kidney stone.

● HOMEOPATHIC CARE

See Cystitis Section and Chapter Five, Colic section.

● HERBAL CARE

Take goldenrod in tincture form three drops three times a day.

Lyme Disease

Lyme disease is spread through ticks by the Borrelia burgdorferi bacteria. (There are other forms of Borrelia infections from ticks and louse including relapsing fever and typhus). Symptoms are normally seen within 30 days of infection. In about 20-30% of cases, there is a red circular rash around bite area. This can be followed with acute aching, joint pains, fever and exhaustion. Secondary symptoms include chronic fatigue, fibromyalgia, weakness, mental confusion and weakness, Bell's Palsy and other neurological issues. Tertiary symptoms include paralysis, multiple sclerosis, mental weakness and imbalance, including psychotic states and heart pathology.

It is prevalent in North America and Europe but can be found worldwide. It was so-named after outbreaks of acute arthritic conditions traced to the tick were found in Old Lyme, Connecticut, USA in the 1970's. Ticks are mostly caught when walking in rural and wooded areas. Ticks have always been carriers of disease but this apparently new strain of Lyme disease has become both an acute and chronic epidemic in recent years. Acute cases are diagnosed through conventional blood tests and treated with antibiotics. However, blood tests will mostly be negative if done before three weeks and after eight weeks from the initial infection. However, if a circular rash forms around a tick bite, called Erythema migrans (EM), then one can assume a bite has occurred and it is possible for it to be infected by the Borrelia bacteria. Not all bites are infectious but given the potential severity of the disease, conventional treatment with antibiotics and also alternative treatment is recommended.

There are many people who suffer chronic consequences of the initial Lyme disease infection and should be treated by a professional homeopath or other health professional. Even when antibiotics are taken for the initial infections, up to 30% of people suffer some form of chronic consequences. That is why it is also important to take homeopathic treatment as well.

Diagnosis of the disease is not always clear and has become a medical controversy due to differing opinions of the disease and the challenge to obtain a positive diagnosis through blood tests. Some doctors now specialize in Lyme disease, yet conventional treatment varies widely but often involves large doses of strong antibiotic therapy, sometimes for years. However, this is not recommended by many medical authorities and the evidence to support long term antibiotic therapy is questionable. There are now various support groups for Lyme disease, some suggesting that a wide range of chronic conditions can be attributable to undiagnosed Lyme disease.

A positive diagnosis of a Borrelia infection by a tick is done by assessing an antibody reaction with either a Western Blot or Elisa test. The tests only indicate that an infection has taken place, not whether you are or will get sick. Also, a negative test does not mean that an infection has not taken place or that the symptoms you are experiencing are from another cause. It could still be Lyme disease. There are more sophisticated tests now (in specialized clinics) to evaluate whether an infection has taken place which can be helpful when a person is sick but nothing is being revealed. However, in the end, it doesn't really matter that much what the tests say. Treatment should be given based on the presenting symptom picture. Doctors and other health therapists who are cognizant of Lyme symptoms should be able to evaluate it based on the history of the symptom picture, although until now, many doctors and therapists have not understood the complexity of the condition and have been unable to give many sufferers an appropriate answer to the mystery of their condition. This is especially when symptoms are in a chronic phase.

From a homeopathic point of view, it can be considered that the original infection of the Borrelia bacteria may have instigated the disease but it then activates a latent susceptibility and general immune deficiency in chronic cases, irrespective of whether the Borrelia is still active or not. Also, even if the bacteria are still active, the long term use of antibiotics can lower the natural immunity of the individual and develop greater tolerance to the antibiotics. Homeopathically, the focus is on the terrain, the individual constitution, not just the precipitating cause - the bacteria. Also, there are known co-infections, (Babesia, Erhlechia, Bartonella) as well as other neurotoxins released through the initial infection that will not be covered by the antibiotics. The impact of these co-infections varies from person to person but is mixed in with the overall symptom picture. Babesia is a parasitic co-infection and Erlechia and Bartonella are bacteria. Babesia infection can look like malaria.

If Lyme disease is diagnosed soon (within a few days) after the bite occurred, then a course of anti-biotics is generally given. (This is a more prophylactic treatment as people are mostly asymptomatic at this point and won't test positive if tested). In some cases, this is enough to deal with it. However, in other cases, it does not work and may even complicate the situation. As mentioned, up to 30% of primary Lyme disease cases continue to have symptoms even after treatment, which mostly look like fibromyalgia and/or chronic fatigue syndrome. *One should still take a homeopathic remedy even if conventional treatment is taken in the first stage and constitutional homeopathic care should be sought if chronic symptoms remain after any treatment taken.* This is especially the case in second and third stages of the disease when conventional treatment can be particularly challenging and questionable in terms of effectiveness.

The first stage of the disease is where there is a raised red rash over the area of the bite, usually within 30 days of the bite. This may be associated with 'flu-like symptoms and aching of the body and fever. It is in situations of acute fever and joint pains that antibiotics can be effective. The second stage develops with more chronic joint, muscle and bone pains, along with great tiredness and weakness. There may also be more acute neurological conditions, like Bell's palsy (one sided facial paralysis), numbness, a lack of coordination, mental fatigue and memory loss. In the third stage, more severe neurological conditions may be seen, resembling multiple sclerosis, Parkinson's disease, severe Epstein Barre, general paresis and paralysis, and also heart pathology. Mentally there may be greater confusion, mood swings, and even psychotic conditions and deep depression. These symptoms may come on years after the initial infection and can be very hard to relate back to the original tick bite. It is only in recent years that this connection has been made to Lyme disease, making diagnosis and treatment all that more difficult.

Lyme disease has similarities with syphilis, with phases of symptom development and neurological and mental symptoms. Also the infection in both cases is a spirochete bacterium, having the shape of a spiral.

● GENERAL CARE

It is important to check for ticks after walking in any rural, wooded area where ticks are found. The whole of New England in the USA is a major source of ticks as are major parts of Europe, especially the Rhineland part of Germany. Any tick that is found should be removed. This is not easy and often the head of the tick can be left in the skin and become infected. Therefore, if possible try and get the tick to let go by itself or if the tick does not come off, take a pair of tweezers and gently remove the whole of the tick. Pull the tick without twisting or pulling suddenly to prevent part of it remaining. If the head does remain, it should be removed by scraping it out. Wash the area well after and use *Calendula* tincture and then cream or other antiseptic lotion, like tea tree oil. It is important to treat the bite homeopathically even if there are no symptoms. At times it has been advised to put heat or a noxious substance onto the tick. The problem can be that it will encourage the tick to expel more bacteria into the body. The best way is to simply pull the tick out with tweezers.

● HOMEOPATHIC CARE

Ledum is the specific remedy for tick bites and should be given both to treat any immediate symptoms after a bite or just as a preventative measure. Symptoms include a 'flu-like ache of any joints, a local swelling of the area affected, with puffiness and coldness to the part and wandering muscular pains of local inflammation to one or more joints.

Kalmia and *Rhododendron* are other homeopathic remedies to be considered if *Ledum* does not work effectively enough after one week. The remedies should be given a minimum of three times a day for a week and then once a day for one more week. *Guajacum* is indicated when the pain is felt mainly in the bones and joints. The joints are often worse from warmth and better from a cold application although they feel worse from cold and damp in general. Pain can extend from the ankles upwards and there can be a contraction feeling in the joints and muscles with a desire to stretch. It can be given if symptoms remain after *Ledum* has been given.

A homeopathic remedy made from the Borrelia bacteria can also be given after a bite to help prevent subsequent infection. It should be given in a 30c or 200c potency once a day for three days and then repeated once a week for 4 weeks. It is not likely to be so helpful on its own for the current attack, more as prevention, but it can help the other remedies work more effectively.

Professional homeopathic and other natural medicine care should be sought when symptoms remain or develop further. It is important to treat the underlying constitution to prevent further symptoms developing. This includes when people are taking long-term antibiotic therapy. The complex and hidden nature of Lyme disease requires a comprehensive approach for which homeopathy and other natural therapies are well suited.

✪ HERBAL CARE

Teasel (*dipsacus*) should be taken as soon as any bite has occurred, both to treat and as a preventative measure. It can be taken as a tincture, one drop in two ounces of water three times a day. If symptoms have already developed and there is much weakness and/or pain, then it may need to be taken more slowly, beginning with one drop on the first day, one drop twice on the second day, one drop thrice on the third day, then each day adding one drop in three separate doses, e.g., (2+1+1) on the fourth, (2+2+1) on the fifth, (2+2+2) on the sixth until on the ninth day it is (3+3+3) drops. This can be taken for one month and then the dose should be reduced again. The dose can always be reduced if there is a strong reaction at any time, as it is not uncommon for there to be a dying off, or detoxifying process, called a Herxheimer reaction.

Cat's claw is another well-known herbal treatment for Lyme symptoms. It has an antibacterial and antiparasitic action. It is one of the main lines of herbal treatment against Lyme disease. Artemesia annua (sweet wormwood) is used when there are symptoms of the co-infection Babesia, which is called Babesiosis.

It is a parasite which occurs with Lyme disease and often with this infection you can feel feverish with great aching in the joints. Dosage will depend on the source and strength of the herbs and should be researched when purchased.

Menstrual Issues, Pregnancy and Menopause

Most menstrual and menopausal problems require more constitutional care as they are mostly chronic in nature. However, in more acute situations or when away, the more immediate symptoms can be treated to give relief. For bleeding problems, also *look at Chapter Three: Accidents, Injuries and Trauma, Hemorrhage and Pain sections.* Acute nausea in pregnancy can be treated as well as threatened miscarriage. The same remedies below apply.

◗ HOMEOPATHIC CARE

Chamomilla is given for excessive cramping pains which feel unbearable and with anger. The pains make one double up, with a need to press strongly into the abdomen.

Magnesium phosphoricum has similar pains, with strong cramping and where pressure and also hot applications and rubbing give relief. The period may have come early with the pains.

Nux vomica is given when there is great sensitivity to all impressions, great irritability and impatience.

Sepia is needed when there is great bearing down pains, as if the uterus is going to come out and you have to sit down. You feel exhausted and irritable. Remedies needed during menopause are often the same as for menstrual and pregnancy issues. ***Pulsatillla***, ***Sepia*** and ***Lachesis*** are important remedies for heat flashes and also excessive bleeding as well as emotional changes at that time. See Nausea section in Chapter Five and remedies specifically for labor in the companion book, *The Natural Medicine Guide for Travel and Home.*

Mouth : Coldsores and Ulcers

COLD SORES (HERPES)

These are herpetic eruptions on the lips, mostly experienced as a lumpy swelling, which can be red and irritating. There may be blistering of the area, with pustules/vesicles. Often these are chronic conditions which come out in times of stress but can also come from exposure to sun, dehydration, other current infections and also for no apparent reason. These are different to canker sores which are ulcerations of the lip and mouth. For some people, this is more of a chronic condition and therefore requires more constitutional treatment. If you have an outbreak of cold sores, do not go into the sun; keep the area moist with lip cream. Take L-Lysine topically and internally. Goldenseal and tree tree, lavender and peppermint oil can be applied to the sore. Wild oregano oil can be used both topically and internally.

◆ HOMEOPATHIC CARE

Rhus tox is given in an intense outbreak when the lips burn and itch intensely, often with vesicles and where there is an achy feeling in the body. If cold sores appear especially on the center of the lower lip and are worse from exposure to the sun or come after an emotional upset, take *Natrum muriaticum*, one tablet three times daily for two days.

Ulcers

These are common conditions which at times are more constitutional in nature and require more chronic treatment. However, they can come due to dietary factors as well as acute stress. Abscesses are different from ulcers as they discharge pus and are often found on the gums. *See Toothache section and Chapter Seven: Skin Conditions, Boils.*

◆ HOMEOPATHIC CARE

Borax is a remedy for for children with small ulcers in the mouth, commonly called aphthae. They are weepy and clingy and dislike being put down. They can have a fear of falling and therefore cling onto their parents. They have a fear of sudden noises. The aphthae can bleed easily and the mouth may have offensive taste and breath.

Mercurius is the other main remedy to consider for mouth ulcers, often associated with an increase in salivation, especially at night, and a peculiar metallic or offensive taste in the mouth. If the ulcers are particular painful, with sharp pains and much salivation and offensive breath and perhaps cracks in the tongue or corner of the mouth, then *Nitric acid* is very good.

🌿 HERBAL CARE

Golden seal tincture gargled in the mouth is effective. Repeat three times daily. Also clove oil can be used and is very soothing.

Sinusitis

Sinusitis is an infection of the sinus cavities, mostly felt in the nose, cheeks and forehead, although it can be felt in the back of the head also. Often it occurs due to an initial cold which leads to a secondary infection. Sometimes it is a chronic condition which mostly requires more constitutional treatment. However, in acute situations it can be effectively treated. *See Fever, Influenza Section.*

⚫ GENERAL CARE

Using a neti pot to clear the sinuses with saline water is an effective way to prevent sinusitis and also to help clear the sinuses of infected mucus. Sometimes this is enough to cure a simple sinusitis. These can be bought at certain pharmacies and health food stores.

💧 HOMEOPATHIC CARE

Kali bichromicum is the most specific remedy for sinusitis when there are symptoms of great pressure in the sinuses, especially felt at the root of the nose and in the cheeks. Often you feel obstructed in the nose but nothing comes out when blowing it, or there is thick, stringy mucus that is hard to detach. There can also be profuse sticky mucus going down the back of the throat.

Belladonna is good when acute sinusitis is attached to a fever and there is heat and throbbing in the sinuses and face, with much congestion.

❂ HERBAL CARE

Golden seal should be taken by holding it in the mouth. Essential oils such as pine, tea tree and/or thyme can be taken as inhalations when mixed with hot water and the steam inhaled.

Teething

Teething is a normal development in a child but often during teething a child can become very upset emotionally and also it can have more general effects for the child. At times a child can get diarrhea when teething.

Chamomilla, Belladonna, Borax, Ipecac, Magnesium phosphoricum and *Silicea* can be thought of. At times it requires constitutional treatment and can be part of other development issues in a child, such as late developing walking or talking and in those cases *Calcarea carbonica* and *Silicea* are two of the main remedies. The child needing *Calcarea carbonica* is more chubby and sweaty, while *Silicea* is more thin, fragile looking and sweaty.

◆ HOMEOPATHIC CARE

Chamomilla. is the first remedy to consider for teething, when the child is easily upset, weepy, irritable and very contrary. Often children want to be picked up and carried and then put down again. Nothing can satisfy them. A child can ask for food and then throw it away. It can drive the parent to distraction.

Borax is needed if the child wants to be carried all the time and has a fear of being put down. If ***Chamomilla*** doesn't work, give ***Borax***. The child may also have apthae (sores) in the mouth.

Ipecac is needed if there is vomiting associated with teething and ***Magnesium phosphoricum*** if there is abdominal cramping.

Throat Conditions

This includes all forms of sore throat, tonsillitis, laryngitis, lost voice etc. Many of the remedies recommended can be found for many other types of infections. A sore throat often comes with other more general symptoms, a fever, a general cold, influenza or bronchitis. However, some people simply get a sore throat once a year, which is relatively mild. Only treat it if it is limiting, painful or it can lead to something worse. One of the most dangerous throat infections is diphtheria but is rarely seen nowadays. If traveling in developing countries, it is possible it would be seen and should be suspected if the sore throat is extremely intense, with fever and chill, difficulty breathing, foul bloody nasal discharge and enlarged lymph glands in the neck. It can be treated with antibiotics. Children can often get sore throats with inflammation of tonsils.

● GENERAL CARE

As with any infection, including colds, keeping warm is important and this is especially the case with throat conditions. Wrap the neck up and drink warm drinks. Sucking lozenges may give relief but don't do it the same time as taking a remedy. Don't strain the voice if the larynx and trachea are affected.

● HOMEOPATHIC CARE

Belladonna is one of the best remedies for simple tonsillitis and throat inflammation when it is sudden, intense and associated with burning and fever. There is an affinity for the right side of the throat. The tongue can look red and shiny.

Hepar sulph and *Mercurius* are two of the best remedies for inflamed throat and tonsillitis when there are sharp, stitching pains in the throat, extending into the ears when swallowing. *Hepar sulph* especially is useful when it feels like a needle or splinter is in the throat and the pain is often better from warm liquids and wrapping up the throat. It is much worse from cold liquids. There may be a hoarse voice. *Mercurius* is needed when there is often an offensive taste in the mouth, mostly metallic, insipid or just bad, with a yellow coating of the tongue. Often there is an increased salivation, even dribbling on the pillow at night. There can be trembling of the tongue when it is protruded.

Phytolacca is a good remedy for simple sore throats, especially when the lymph glands of the neck are swollen and tender, for which *Mercurius* is also indicated. Tonsils are swollen and red, and the neck is stiff. Symptoms are often better when cold drinks are taken and become worse from warmth.

Lachesis is useful when the left side of the throat is mostly affected, and there is a feeling of a lump in the throat. There is difficulty in swallowing, especially liquids, whereas solids are easier.

Arum tryphillum is used when there is great rawness of the throat with a lost voice, the pain worse from coughing or clearing the throat. *Rhus tox* is good for a simple lost voice from using the voice too much or exposure to cold weather. *Argentum nitricum* is useful when you lose your voice before having to perform or give a talk, a form of anticipatory anxiety.

NOTE It is not always easy to find the correct remedy. Try one and if it does not work in one to two days, try another. If it is a simple sore throat with no discernible symptoms, try *Phytolacca* first and follow with *Mercurius* if needed.

Toothache

A toothache always needs to be checked with a dentist to find out the reason for the pain. However, using homeopathic remedies can relieve the pain and at times deal with the whole situation. Be careful when having dental work in places where the quality cannot be guaranteed. When you have an abscess of the gums, it may be due to a simple infection, which can happen when traveling and when coming across more unusual bacteria. It can also indicate a deeper problem in the roots of the teeth. If that is so, dentists mostly will recommend a root canal. However, if traveling, it is best to treat the infection, either with antibiotics and or homeopathic remedies and after that get the tooth looked at when you get home. Some dentists can want to do root canals very quickly when perhaps the body will take care of the problem itself. If you really do need a root canal, the body will tell you as the abscess or pain will come back. It is often not an emergency and the situation should be reviewed once the infection is cleared up. This is both when traveling and when at home. Find a dentist you can really trust! *See Chapter Three: Accidents, Injuries and Trauma, Pain.*

● **GENERAL CARE**

Taking pain killers as necessary and also using cloves to help to numb the area can help. Do not take at the same time as a homeopathic remedy as it may antidote the remedy. If there is an abscess in the gums, keep the mouth very clean. Gargle with salt water and also use essential oils such as wintergreen, peppermint, oregano and eucalpytus as well as taking cloves.

◆ **HOMEOPATHIC CARE**

Homeopathy can work quickly to relieve the pain if the underlying problem is not severe. The pain will be relieved in minutes to a couple of hours, depending on the severity of the pain.

Chamomilla is the first remedy for teething children who are irritable and capricious and who have colic and/or diarrhea from teething. It can also be used for general tooth pain.

Coffea is the first remedy to consider for severe pain. There is great sensitivity in the teeth, which is worse from all stimulation, noises etc. The pain is worse from touch and chewing and better from ice water in the mouth. You are not able to sleep because of the pain. Use *Nux vomica* when there is great pain with sensitivity to all stimuli and a feeling of great irritability with the pain. Also consider *Magnesium phosphoricum* for teething and teeth pains which are better from warmth and pressure.

Hepar sulph, *Mercurius* and *Silicea* are given for abscess es of the gums, similar to when given for abscesses of the skin. *Hepar sulph* is needed for very painful abscesses with sharp, stitching pains; *Mercurius* when there is a painful abscess, with increased saliva and at times a foul, or metallic taste in the mouth. There may be swelling of the cheek on the affected side. *Silicea* is often needed if the problem recurs and if there is discharge from the absecess.

Staphysagria is also useful for abscesses when it recurs and also when there is decaying of the roots or crown of the teeth, and blackening of the teeth. *Hekla lava* is indicated when there is hard swelling of the jaw with a large abscess. *See Chapter Seven: Skin Conditions, Boils.*

COMBINATION STRATEGY If you are not sure which remedy is needed, mix one tablet of *Hepar sulph* and *Mercurius* into two to four ounces of water and take one tsp. three to five times daily.

Chapter Seven
Skin Conditions

There are many skin conditions, some of which accompany other illnesses mentioned in the book and need to be studied with those conditions. When traveling some conditions are seen that are due to a combination of being in intense heat or from poor hygiene, dirty hotels etc. These are either fungal or parasite infections. Hygiene is the key to prevention, but at times they can't be avoided. When traveling, the skin can take a hammering, from too much sun, with difficulties in hygiene, the feet drying out leading to cracking and pain, and various skin infections that easily come from scratches and slight wounds. Take a good soap with you, ideally a liquid soap that is easily portable. Soaps in more basic areas are often not nice and can cause local allergic reactions.

● **GENERAL CARE**

Maintaining good skin is important. Using a ripe avocado is one natural way to nourish the skin, mashing up the avocado and applying immediately. It can be left for hours or overnight. Using good oil on the skin may help. Coconut oil and other vegetable oils can be used. Clean your feet regularly and rub rough skin off around the heel to prevent drying and cracking and apply oil. For irritating skin conditions of all sorts, putting raw cabbage on the affected area can relieve. This is useful especially for children who are itching intensely at irritated parts. Loosely bandage the cabbage to the irritated part and change daily. Ensure any cuts, abrasions and other wounds are cleaned well and ideally covered for 2-3 days.

Animals: Lice, Fleas and Bedbugs

Lice, fleas and bedbugs are one of the unfortunate consequences of travel and of sleeping in infected beds all over the world. Lice most commonly occur due to poor hygiene and can be more easily avoided. The most commonly seen are head lice, often afflicting children and easily spread. Lice can also be found in the groin and pubic region and are known as crabs. Body lice can be carriers of diseases such as typhus and relapsing fever. Typhus used to be an epidemic disease in times of war and extreme hardship, e.g., prisons and concentration camps. Millions in human history have died as a result of the bacterial infection from lice but in modern times and when traveling, it is generally not seen. Body lice can be spread easily from one person to another and pubic lice through sex. Head lice do not carry these diseases. Head lice are recognized by their nits, pale little balls often seen in the margins of the hair, especially the neck. They are difficult to remove. These nits should be removed, either with a nit comb or even by shaving the head.

● GENERAL CARE

Using coconut oil on the head after washing can help remove the nits. Tea tree oil can also be used to help kill the nits. One problem commonly found is that although the lice can be removed, enough nits remain to re-infect the person, so all nits have to be removed. Treatment needs to be done for at least one week to prevent re-infection. Body lice can be treated in a similar way, using tea tree oil mixed with bathing water and washed onto the skin. Fleas and bed bugs are also common, bed bugs being commonly found in unclean hotels and even in higher class places all over the world. With bed bugs, washing all infected clothing and linens is essential.

● HOMEOPATHIC CARE

Staphysagria is given for bites for itching, irritating and painful bites and also be used for head lice. Take 3 times daily for 3 days.

● HERBAL CARE

Tea tree oil can be used to help with bites and also to prevent being bitten. Other sprays such as pyrethrum can be used.

Boils and Abscesses

Boils are often caused by a bacterial infection, often affecting a hair follicle or due to broken skin becoming infected. If left untreated, they can either erupt or become re-absorbed into the body. A carbuncle is a large boil which is abscessing, often with more than one opening, draining pus onto the skin. The same remedies are needed as with a boil, but it needs to be kept very clean to prevent further infection. A bad carbuncle may need professional medical attention to see what underlying condition may be the primary cause. Recurrent boils or abscesses can also require constitutional treatment once the acute symptoms are controlled.

Abscesses may develop from a boil or be an expression on the skin of a deeper infection in the body, the abscess being a vent for the infection. Once an abscess has burst, it is important to keep it clean and to give appropriate remedies for the abscess and the underlying infection. Abscesses also occur on the gums of the mouth, often due to an underlying infection of the roots of the teeth. The same remedies described below can be used.

● GENERAL CARE

Do not burst a boil. Let it take its own course. Once it has burst, keep clean, wash in warm water and use *Calendula* tincture (diluted in some water). Alternatively use *Echinacea* tincture. Ensure the water is boiled first.

◆ HOMEOPATHIC CARE

Hepar sulph is needed when the boils/abscesses have a sharp, stitching pain and are much worse for touch and cold air. It can feel as though there is a splinter there. *Silicea* is the other remedy for abscesses or boils that don't heal quickly. Both are good remedies for abscesses of the gums. *Silicea* can follow *Hepar sulph* if that remedy doesn't complete the situation and it is good to help finally heal a chronic abscess that isn't healing fully. These are the two main remedies when the boil or abscess is threatening to burst and needs either to be reabsorbed or brought to the surface.

Hekla lava is also a good remedy for abscesses in the gums when the other remedies don't work and when the abscess is hard and the jaw is swollen and painful. (This remedy was found when an English doctor noticed that cows feeding on grass around Mt Hekla in Iceland developed bony growths on their jaws).

Belladonna is needed if the boil is very inflamed and burning with redness and pressure and it comes on very quickly then the remedy needed. There is often great heat and/or stinging.

Lachesis is needed once it has become an abscess and there is burning and becoming a purple color and looks as if it is becoming infected, then. There may be throbbing and discharge of thin, bloody pus.

Tarentula cubensis can be given if the boil threatens to turn into a carbuncle and become more deeply infected, with great burning, then.

Pyrogen can be given if an abscess has developed into a more general systemic infection with classic symptoms of blood poisoning – fever, chill, restlessness, achiness of the body, a rapid pulse but with low temperature, but medical attention should be sought as well.

🌿 HERBAL CARE

Make a clay pack as for bites. Take *Echinacea* tincture, ten drops per hour for four to six hours. Repeat daily for three to five days. Make a hot compress using two drops of tea tree and lavender oil and apply to the area. Also apply neat lavender to the area.

Chilblains

Chilblains are due to a problem with the blood flow to the extremities and exposure to cold weather. A contraction of veins or just bad circulation made worse in the cold creates congestion of blood in the exposed part leading to swelling, itching, redness and burning. It is not a very serious condition and some people are more inclined to get them than others.

⬤ GENERAL CARE

Avoid allowing extremities to become overexposed to the cold. If already afflicted, do not expose to intense heat, but gradually warm the part. The most likely parts affected are the toes, fingers, ears and nose. Rub tea tree oil onto the inflamed parts.

🌢 HOMEOPATHIC CARE

Agaricus is the most specific remedy to give, similar to that of frostbite. *Pulsatilla* is useful when the itching is much worse from the heat, which is often the case and is more often needed as a constitutional remedy for the condition.

Fungal Infections

There are various forms of fungus (commonly called tinea), from one that affects the crotch area (crotch itch or dhobie itch) and classic ringworm (which is a fungal eruption creating round patterns of raised, red skin). It can also occur on the scalp, creating bald patches, and is mainly seen in children. In another form of skin fungus - tinea versicolor - one sees blotches of skin discoloration which look lighter or at times darker than the rest of the skin. Another fungus is commonly known as athletes' foot. This latter condition is extremely common, highly infectious and difficult to get rid of. One needs to treat it for up to one month continually and even then it can tend to return.

Another common fungal condition is candida. It can be found all over the body and often begins with little red dots that gets more red, raised and angry and gradually spread from the original outbreak. It is mostly found in the warm areas of the body, the armpits, crotch and under the breasts. It is often the cause of diaper rash in babies or a secondary infection. Candida is also found in the genital region of women and also in the nipples of breast feeding women. Thrush is a form of candida commonly found in the mouths of babies. Candida albicans is a form of candida often found in the digestive tract and also the respiratory tract and genitalia. They are normally found there but at times they greatly increase in number, leading to local and systemic symptoms. It has been speculated in recent years that when people have chronic candida infections in the body it lead to other more chronic problems and much has been written about candida diets and other therapies to purge the candida from the body. In a healthy body, fungi should not be able to prosper. However, the abuse of antibiotics for generations, including the amount in the food supply, along with other external factors may be one reason why there has been a huge increase in fungal conditions of all sorts in recent years. For example, in those who are immune deficient, such as people who are HIV positive it is often seen that systemic fungal infections are found along with other conditions.

● GENERAL CARE

Keep the skin well-washed and in cases where the groin is affected, allow as much air as possible. There are many different natural external topical treatments that can be used. Some may work better than others, depending on the person and also the severity of the infection. Eat very little or no sugar. Even cut down on fruits to lower the amount of sugar in the system. Fungi thrive on sugar. Conventional anti-fungal treatments can be used on the skin if necessary.

◆ HOMEOPATHIC CARE

Borax and *Mercurius*. are useful for babies with thrush. *See Chapter Six: Mouth ulcers.* For general thrush, more constitutional care is needed but local herbal applications can be effective as well as changing habits, such as diet and hygiene measures. For diaper rash, *Belladonna*, *Chamomilla* and *Rhus tox* are often needed.

Dulcamara is used for ringworm, especially on the scalp with thick crusts, moist and dry, and round patches of hair loss, giving it three times daily for up to one week. Other more chronic based remedies are *Calcarea carbonica*, *Graphites* and *Sulphur*. The first is used in young children, who are generally overweight and sweaty, especially about the head, and where the whole head may be covered with crusts. In *Graphites*, there is oozing of honey like liquid which then dries up and in *Sulphur*, there is insufferable itching, especially when they get warm.

🍃 HERBAL CARE

Tea tree oil and lavender are used to treat many types of tinea. They can be mixed with a neutral oil, like olive or almond oil and put onto the affected parts after washing. For tinea versicolor, using apple cider vinegar can work. Tea tree oil or garlic oil can be used for athlete's foot. Neem oil can also be used for all types of fungal infections, including vaginal candida, where it can be mixed with yoghurt or olive oil.

Hives

Hives are a type of urticarial eruption, often with swelling, redness, bumps and itching of the skin. It can come from an allergic reaction, usually to food, e.g., shellfish or some external irritant, e.g., pollen, or it can come from being stressed. The body releases too much histamine, resulting in a skin eruption. Hives can come from overexposure to the sun or simply due to sensitivity to the sun. This sensitivity can be induced by taking medications and other products, including using sun block! If possible, stop taking any offending product but even then it can take a while for any allergic reaction to subside. *See Chapter Six: Allergies section.*

◆ HOMEOPATHIC CARE

Apis is one of the first remedies for hives when there is stinging, burning and redness of the skin, associated mostly with a general allergic reaction to some external stimuli, e.g., shellfish. Often there is swelling with the redness and may be seen on the face, especially around the eyes.

Urtica urens is the other major remedy for hives which are caused by shellfish and has similar symptoms, especially great stinging of the skin.

Rhus tox is the other major remedy for hives and looks very similar to *Apis*. All three remedies can be combined if necessary.

Impetigo

One other common condition found especially in children is the highly infectious bacterial disease, impetigo. It is mostly found on the face and consists of itchy, crusty eruptions, at times oozing sticky moisture. As it is infectious and can spread to other children quickly, antibiotic therapy is mostly given. It is good to keep your child away from others if he/she is affected and treat either with both homeopathy and conventional medicine.

◆ HOMEOPATHIC CARE

Antimonium crudum is one of the most important remedies for impetigo. There are crusty thick eruptions, both dry and moist and are found anywhere on the body, but especially the face. Mentally, children are often cross, peevish and averse to being looked at.

Rhus tox is another remedy to consider when there are eruptions rather like shingles. *Mezereum* can also be given for impetigo.

Croton tiglium is one other remedy to think of when there are thick, rough, crusty eruptions which burst. The skin can feel thick and rough. *Dulcamara* is useful when the eruptions are thick, crusty and become moist and perhaps have come on after exposure to cold and damp. *See Shingles Section.*

COMBINATION STRATEGY If you do not know which remedy to choose, put one tablet of all the remedies (or which ones you have access to) into four ounces of water, and give one tsp. three times daily for five to seven days. Stop giving it if symptoms either get better or worse.

Poison Oak/Ivy

This is an allergic skin condition due to exposure to various forms of the plant species of poison ivy or poison oak (*Rhus toxicodendrum*, *Rhus radicans*, *Rhus diversiloba*, etc.). It is very common in North America and is found in most rural and wooded areas. Some people are highly allergic and will have a strong local and systemic reaction, affecting all parts of the body, including the genitalia and face, and even the throat. Other people seem virtually immune to it. Often it happens that a dog which has been walking in the woods will spread the resin from the plant to humans. If there is any suspicion of exposure, the skin must be washed very well, along with clothing, and products used to ensure that all the oil is off the body. Many people say different things work for them. Just a small amount on one part of the body can spread to other parts and eruptions will appear in one place and then another and then another. The rash can last from ten days to about three weeks although it can be longer in sensitive people.

Symptoms consist of blistery eruptions, redness, heat and great itching. The skin can swell, becoming very painful and it can affect all parts of the body. It can be a tormenting condition for those who are sensitive. Conventional treatment begins with antihistamines and calamine and moves to systemic steroids, either tablets or injections if very serious. Even then, it can take a while for real relief to settle in.

◆ HOMEOPATHIC CARE

Rhus tox (homeopathic poison ivy) is given first if it is suspected that infection with poison oak or ivy has taken place. It is best to take one tablet three times daily for three days. If symptoms develop, continue this remedy to see if it helps. If it doesn't, a combination strategy should be employed, taking the following remedies: *Anacardium*, *Arsenicum album* and *Croton tiglium*. One tablet of each should be mixed in water and one tsp. taken four times daily for three to five days. Also *Rhus diversoloba* (another remedy from the same botanical family) can be tried if *Rhus tox* doesn't work or in combination with it in the beginning.

NOTE This is not easy to treat and there may be other indicated remedies. Professional homeopathic advice is recommended if relief is not found.

Scabies

Scabies is a common skin affection due to the scabies mite, a parasite that bores into the skin, causing immense itchiness. It is difficult to see but often one may see little black points or lines between the fingers or in the creases of the skin. Itching is often much worse at night and from the heat. It is highly infectious and easily caught by contact with others or by using the same bedding. The skin may blister or form small itchy lumps in various parts of the body. If one person has it, the whole family should be treated.

● **GENERAL CARE**

All clothing and bedding must be thoroughly washed and repeated even daily for one week. The mites are very tenacious. You can take one cup of kerosene/paraffin and mix with one cup of vegetable oil and apply twice daily for two days after washing, to all areas affected. Neem oil can also be used.

● **HOMEOPATHIC CARE**

Sulphur is a specific remedy for this condition and should be taken three times a day for up to seven days. Stop the remedy if relief of the itching is felt or if the itching gets much worse after the remedy.

Arsenicum album is given if there is burning of the skin with great restlessness and anxiety. If the condition remains persistent, consider giving *Psorinum* for up to five days. It is a nosode made from scabies.

🖊 HERBAL CARE

Use tea tree oil or lavender on the itchiest parts of the skin.

Shingles (Herpes Zoster)

Shingles is a viral condition affecting the skin and is connected to the chicken pox virus. It creates extremely painful swelling and blisters, irritating superficial nerves near the skin. It can affect any part of the body, including the face and also the torso and tends to often occur in one particular place. It most prominently affects elderly people and those under severe stress or suffering other immune compromised diseases such as AIDS. At times, the pain is the first symptom to occur before the rash appears. If untreated, it can last for weeks. Also, even after treatment, some people experience post herpetic neuralgia where areas of the skin remain inflamed. Conventional treatment involves pain relief and anti-viral drugs but it is not always that effective. However, it is important to give some pain relief medicine when it is very intense.

♦ HOMEOPATHIC CARE

Rhus tox is the first remedy to consider for shingles. It has the classic eruption of blisters (vesicles) which are burning, itching and with sharp stitching pains. The skin can look and feel thick. The eruptions may be dry, crusty and moist. The pains can be better for warm applications and if bad, one can feel chilled, as if cold water is being thrown over the body.

Mezereum can be given if *Rhus tox* doesn't work, especially if it affects one side of the face only. The blisters may ooze sticky moisture and then form thick crusts. Symptoms are better in the cool, open air.

Ranunculus bulbosa is given when pains are extreme, with shooting, stitching pains which can even induce tears. Eruptions may be especially on the chest, making it difficult to breathe and become much worse from any touch.

NOTE Skin conditions are not always easy to treat homeopathically. Finding the exact picture can be difficult. If *Rhus tox* doesn't work, then go to one of the other remedies or combine them both. If the pain is severe, then one should expect some relief in the pain within twelve hours to one day but it will take some days before new eruptions stop coming. Keep giving the remedy until significant relief is achieved. If there is some improvement over one week but then no further improvement is seen, give *Graphites*, one tablet four times a day for three to five days. *Mercurius* can also be considered if the eruptions are very painful and itch at night and *Arsenicum album* if there is despair from pain. Also, professional medical care may be needed, especially in elderly people and where the eyes are affected.

Ulcers

Skin ulcers are common in tropical climates and most commonly affect people below the knee, especially around the foot if the foot is mostly exposed through wearing flip-flops all the time. It often begins from a minor injury to the skin, when the skin is broken, even from scratching a bite or pimple and a secondary bacterial infection takes place. Gradually or at times quite suddenly the ulcer spreads and can become painful, and an offensive or watery discharge can be seen. Often these ulcers will eventually resolve but it is imperative to take good care of the wound to aid the healing and prevent complication. More serious complications involve infection of the bone, or a more systemic blood infection affecting the whole body and the development of much fibrous scar tissue, preventing healing. Therefore, especially when traveling, it is imperative to look after the wound, keep it clean and if very bad, to stop traveling until some healing has taken place. Ulcers can also come from a staphylococcal bacterial infection in the blood, and this can lead to recurrent ulcers on the skin, beginning as a small boil and quickly spreading into a large ulcer. They can take a long time to heal. One needs to be careful with a staphylococcal infection that it does not lead to a more general septic condition of the body. Medical intervention can be necessary.

● GENERAL CARE

An ulcer should be kept clean. It should be washed with clean, disinfected water, with some drops of *Calendula* lotion in a ratio of 1:10 approximately. Conventional antiseptic like hydrogen peroxide is also good. Any dead skin should be removed. If the wound is relatively superficial without pus formation, an oil based *Calendula* lotion can be used on the ulcer and then covered with a non-adhesive dressing or gauze. It is important that the dressing does not stick to the ulcer, which would prevent new skin from forming when the dressing is removed.

If the ulcer is deeper and there is pus formation, then *Calendula* solution should be mixed with some water (ratio of 1:10) and a dressing soaked in this solution should be put onto the ulcer. The dressing should always be wet and the *Calendula* mixture can be sprayed onto the dressing to keep it moist. Change the dressing daily. Clear plastic or a plastic bag can be used to cover the dressing to keep it moist. This should be continued until the infection is clean. If *Calendula* is not available use other local antiseptic lotions, such as hydrogen peroxide, isopropyl alcohol or iodine initially. These have also been counter indicated in superficial wounds due to their tendency to increase scar tissue and healing time. The most important thing is to initially clean the wound, using these or other products. Once the ulcer is clean, try and leave it exposed to the air, using only a small amount of calendula cream. If on the foot or lower leg, do not walk anymore than absolutely necessary. However if there is a need to travel the ulcer should be bandaged as described above.

Manuka honey or other honey is a strong antibacterial to treat ulcers and also burns. It can be used alongside *Calendula* to help heal the ulcer at both the initial stage of pus formation and for secondary healing. Tea tree oil can be used similarly.

◆ HOMEOPATHIC CARE

Arsenicum album is needed for ulcers with great burning but which may feel better from warm application. There can be anxiety and restlessness with the ulcer and it is for infected ulcers with offensive, burning discharges.

Carbo vegetabalis is indicated for ulcers that are burning but which also can feel cold, and it is good for infected ulcers in which the skin is blue.

Lachesis is needed for infected ulcers with a bluish/purple color and which are very sensitive to touch. The ulcer looks as though it is becoming very infected. It is the first remedy to think of ulcers which come from a bite of a poisonous animal.

Mercurius is for ulcers with ragged edges with an offensive yellow discharge, which bleeds easily and the margins look like raw meat.

COMBINATION STRATEGY If in doubt, combine one tablet of *Mercurius*, *Arsenicum album*, *Carbo veg* and *Lachesis* in a glass of water and take one tsp. four times a day for three to five days.

Chapter Eight
Tropical Diseases

Most of these diseases are fairly rare for most travelers. Malaria is the most common disease acquired by travelers, follwed by dengue fever and typhoid fever. Bilharzia is also a common and serious condition found in many tropical areas and needs to be paid attention to. Yellow fever is rarely seen and a vaccine is required for travel to Sub-Saharan Africa and the Amazonia region of Brazil. This is the only mandatory vaccine for any travel. However, it is only likely to be checked when entering from countries where yellow fever is found and not when entering via air from Europe or North America etc. For most of these diseases if homeopathic treatment is suitable, remedies are recommended or are referred to other relevant chapters, especially *Chapter Six: Common Infections* as fevers are a common aspect of many of these diseases.

Disease Risks for Travelers
Prevention and Treatment

AFRICAN SLEEPING SICKNESS (HUMAN AFRICAN TRYPANOSOMIASIS) Fairly Low Risk

- Found in Sub-Saharan Africa (West, Central and East Africa).
- Parasite spread by tsetse fly. In West Africa, found mainly around rivers and water. In East Africa, found around drier bush land.
- Prevent being bitten. Using insect repellants is important. Conventional treatment is available.

BILHARZIA (SCHISTOSOMIASIS) High Risk

- Endemic throughout the world. Especially seen in Sub-Saharan Africa, The Nile region of Egypt, South America, The Caribbean, China, Philippines and Japan.
- A worm which infects an aquatic snail found in fresh water areas and spreads to humans. All fresh water, e.g., lakes, rivers, streams is suspect.
- If in fresh water, wear clothes or boots, wet suits etc. Rub off well if getting wet. Be careful swimming in lakes. Check out disease incidence. Conventional treatment is available.

CHAGAS DISEASE (AMERICAN TRYPTOMANIASIS)
Low Risk

- Found mostly in rural areas of Central and South America.
- A parasite spread through the bite of an insect.
- Be careful if staying in homes of poor people in rural areas. Conventional treatment works well in acute phase, less well in chronic phases.

CHOLERA Low Risk

- Endemic in areas of extremely poor hygiene and trauma due to war. More seen in Africa, the Indian subcontinent and South East Asia.
- A bacterial infection spread through contaminated food and water.
- Avoid areas of epidemic if possible and ensure food and water is clean. Conventional treatment is effective if done early.
- Vaccine available but only 50-60% effective.

DENGUE FEVER Medium Risk

- Endemic in Sub-Saharan Africa, South East Asia, India, the Caribbean and Central and South America. Found more in urban areas.
- A viral infection caught from mosquitoes.

- Avoiding being bitten by mosquitoes. Use of repellants, nets and clothing. Conventional treatment not available.

MALARIA High Risk

- Endemic in all tropical areas, especially Sub-Saharan Africa, South East Asia and Amazonia of South America.
- A parasitic infection caught from mosquitoes.
- Avoiding being bitten by mosquitoes. Use of conventional malaria prophylactics. Conventional treatment is available.

TYPHOID Medium Risk

- Endemic in most tropical and sub tropical areas of the world, especially Africa, India, most of Asia and Central and South America.
- A bacterium caught from contaminated food and water.
- Ensuring food and water eaten is clean by eating in good places and not drinking contaminated water. Conventional treatment available.

African Sleeping Sickness
(Human African Trypanosomiasis)

ONSET Symptoms can come on slowly. Initial symptoms
may be absent and only months or years later will symptoms
develop. Medical intervention is crucial.

KEY SYMPTOMS Fever. Head and body aches, coming and
going. Swelling of lymph nodes. Neurological problems,
tremors, convulsions, lack of coordination. Lethargy, sleepiness.
Character change, argumentative, fitful, indifference.

This is known as sleeping sickness and is a parasitic disease spread by
the tsetse fly. It is found mainly in rural areas of Sub-Saharan Africa
and most prominent sleeping sickness cases are found in West,
Central and East Africa. Over sixty million people are affected.
In West Africa, the tsetse flies are found mainly around rivers and
other watery areas. In East Africa, they are found more in drier bush
land areas. Travelers are not that likely to come across this condition
unless some time is spent in such areas. In urban areas, there is no
real problem. Even in rural areas, infection rates vary widely in a
similar geographical area. It is worth investigating this if time is to
be spent in such areas. It can also be spread from mother to child,
from blood transfusions and perhaps through sexual transmission.

The West and Central African variety can begin very slowly
and without any noticeable symptoms for months and even years.
However, within some weeks of infection, there may be symptoms
of fever, headache, body aches etc., but which can come and go,

with periods of well-being in between. There may be swelling of the liver and spleen and much swelling of lymph nodes in the body. There may develop more serious symptoms at this point and medical intervention is crucial. In some cases, these symptoms will be absent and the first real signs will be problems in the central nervous system, with problems walking, tremors, convulsions etc. The sleeping sickness symptoms are seen in this phase, often with great lethargy. Prior to this there may be some character changes, with fitful, argumentative behavior and indifference. This may occur even years after initial infection, so if a person has spent any lengths of time in areas of infection and then suddenly develops behavioral or neurological conditions, this should be considered.

The East African variety tends to produce a more acute picture earlier on. Symptoms will include a local red, hot swelling around the area of the bite within days followed between one to three weeks later with symptoms of fever and lymphatic swellings described above. Again, medical diagnosis and treatment is crucial as it can lead to death within a number of weeks up to one year after infection. In the West African variety, death can occur over two to three years after initial infection.

● GENERAL CARE

Prevention of being bitten is important. Insect repellants should be used as needed and also pyrethrum spray can be used.
See www.thenaturalmedicineguide.com for prevention information.

◆ HOMEOPATHIC CARE

Professional care is ideally needed.
See Chapter Seven: Common Conditions, Fever and Influenza.

Bilharzia
(Schistosomiasis).

ONSET Nothing may be seen for up to two years from infection.
There may be some initial skin irritation, but often nothing is
noticed. In other cases, symptoms of fever, diarrhea, cough, skin
irritation are seen within 8 weeks.
KEY SYMPTOMS Blood in urine. Inflammation of bladder,
prostate and genitalia. Fever, malaise, diarrhea, skin rash, cough.
Dysentery, blood and mucus in bowel. Liver and spleen enlarged.

Bilharzia is one of the most common serious diseases in certain
regions of the world, predominantly Africa, South America and
Asia. Only malaria has more impact on affected societies.

There are four or five varieties, each affecting different organs
although the symptom pictures may be similar. It is an endemic
condition throughout the world caused by a worm called
Schistosomes which infect an aquatic snail found in fresh water areas.
Once they leave the snail they infect the human host and from there,
move to various organs of the body, causing acute and potentially
serious chronic consequences. Therefore, the most important thing
for the traveler is to avoid fresh water in those regions, including

lakes, rivers and ponds, etc., any standing water in which snails may exist. It can be highly infectious and slight exposure to the water, like wading across a stream, may cause infection. Prevention is the best course. Do not swim in open fresh water, do not expose parts of the body to the water; avoid dammed water and if exposed, dry off and change clothes as quickly as possible. Do not stay wet and wear clothing or a wet suit to cross bodies of water.

One form of the disease affects the urinary organs, including the kidney, the prostate and the uterus. This form of bilharzia is found mainly in most of Africa and especially in the Nile region of Egypt. The incubation period after initial infection may take up to two years to manifest, making the initial diagnosis difficult. There may be some mild initial itching of the skin after infection, but little more. The first symptoms to be seen may be blood in the urine, especially at the end of urination, and then may develop into cystitis, kidney stones, prostate and uterine infection and even cancer of organs such as the bladder.

Other forms of the disease primarily affect the bowel and the liver. These forms are found in Africa and also in South America (especially the North East of Brazil), parts of the Caribbean, China, Japan and the Philippines. These forms may be more lethal than the first. Symptoms develop more quickly, up to eight weeks after infection, with the onset of a fever, general malaise, diarrhea, a generalized skin rash and cough. At this point, only a blood test will reveal the nature of the disease as it can look like many other conditions, especially malaria. After the fever goes, bowel symptoms can begin with dysentery, with blood and mucus in the stool. From there, the liver and spleen may become enlarged and kidney function begins to fail, leading to heart failure.

In another form of the disease, the initial skin condition may be very intense and the subsequent fever also very intense. There will also be blood in the stool and enlargement of the liver and spleen and there can be great hard swelling of the abdomen. There may be significant amounts of blood in the stool.

● HOMEOPATHIC CARE

This is best treated professionally and it is imperative that a diagnosis is made to confirm the cause of the symptoms. However, if one is traveling and self-treatment is necessary, the following remedies can be considered:

Antimonium tart is good if there are symptoms of great weakness, breathlessness and profound drowsiness. The local bladder or other symptoms are less significant here but may be seen.

China has great weakness, and also has abdominal symptoms such as bloating, lack of appetite and loose stools creating exhaustion. *See Chapter Five: Digestive Conditions, Dysentery and Indigestion sections*. There may be blood in the stool.

Terebinthina is a specific remedy if the main symptom is bleeding from the bladder and also for great burning in the bladder, prostate and/or uterine area. It has abdominal bloating, dysentery and even colitis symptoms. Much bleeding is the key symptom along with burning.

Chagas Disease
(American Trypanosomiasis)

ONSET Often very slow. Initial infection as a child and only as an adult do symptoms develop. In children, there may be a boil developing 1-4 weeks after bite. Then fever comes 1-2 weeks later.

KEY SYMPTOMS In children, they may have a bite, becoming a boil, lasting for months. Conjunctivitis, with swelling of lymph glands. Sudden, intense fever, lasting weeks, and swelling of liver and spleen. Inflammation of brain and heart. In adult, symptoms of heart disease, tendency to strokes, general weakness and digestive problems.

This is a parasitic infection due to the bite of an insect and is found in rural areas of Central and South America. It is a very common disease, found in both acute and long term chronic phases, affecting up to eleven million people, most of who don't know they are infected. Most urban travelers are unlikely to see this disease even though it is quite widespread throughout the region. For most people after infection, there is no apparent illness and the disease remains dormant for many years until the person is an adult in their twenties or thirties. If symptoms do appear in the initial phase and this is mostly with children, there may be skin sensitivity around the area of the bite, resembling a boil, which will last for months. If the point of infection is the eye, then a swelling of the upper and lower eyelids takes place with conjunctivitis and swelling of the lymph glands under the jaw on the affected side. (There is a tendency to bite the cheeks of the face, hence the term 'kissing bugs' is given to the insect. They are also called 'assassin bugs'). Around one week after this, a sudden and intense fever may arise and continue even for weeks. There can be further complications with swelling of the liver and spleen and in very severe cases, heart and brain inflammation, often leading to death. However, the majorities of people do survive this attack but are then prone to serious complications many years later, such as heart weakness, strokes, digestive problems and intellectual weakness.

◆ HOMEOPATHIC CARE

In the acute phase, a remedy must be chosen on the symptom picture. **Ledum**, one tablet three times daily for one week is an obvious one to begin for the affect of the bite, but other remedies for the fever must be considered. In the chronic phase, constitutional care must be sought, along with other medical options.
See Chapter Six Common Conditions, Fever and Influenza sections.

Cholera

ONSET Symptoms come on 2-7 days after infection with sudden attack of diarrhea.
KEY SYMPTOMS Sudden onset of violent diarrhea, very copious rice water and mostly painless. Intense vomiting, chill, cramping and spasms in intestines and throughout body.

Cholera is a bacterial disease and is spread through contaminated water and food. Certain people can be carriers of the disease and once infected, the incubation period is normally between two to seven days. Characteristically, there is a sudden onset of violent diarrhea, which becomes extremely copious, like rice water, and is painless. Often there is projectile vomiting, the great risk being a serious lack of fluids in the body, which if not replaced can lead to kidney failure and death. Therefore, the key to any treatment is rehydration. If possible this is done intravenously but if in remote areas and where no medical help is available, oral rehydration has to suffice. However, homeopathic medicines can be crucial to help the body recover and in cholera epidemics of the nineteenth century, homeopathy showed remarkable successes. In many cases, one may be infected by the cholera bacteria but show very mild symptoms which will not need much treatment. *See Chapter Five: Digestive Conditions, Diarrhea section.*

◆ HOMEOPATHIC CARE

Arsenicum album is the first remedy to consider is. At this stage you may not even know it is cholera and often it will simply get better and you won't know it was a cholera infection. Not all cholera becomes life threatening and if you remain hydrated and are strong, it does not need to become serious. However, the symptoms you may feel will be nausea, vomiting and often diarrhea, all at the same time. There can be great weakness, restlessness and chilliness.

Veratrum album may be needed if *Arsenicum album* doesn't work and if you have profuse cold perspiration on the forehead.

Camphor is needed if there is a great icy coldness of the body yet do not want to be covered and there is anxiety and even despair, along with some cramping. *Cuprum* should be taken if the cramping becomes really intense in any part of the body.

COMBINATION STRATEGY You can combine one or more of the remedies together in water and give one tsp. every hour until some relief.

Dengue Fever

ONSET Symptoms develop between 2-14 days from infection.
KEY SYMPTOMS Sudden onset of fever, aching and crippling bone and joint pains. Severe headache. It looks similar to malaria and yellow fever and can often be confused in initial stages.

Dengue fever is a viral infection spread through mosquito bites. These mosquitoes are often found near human habitation and therefore dengue often occurs in more urban areas. It is found predominantly in Africa, South-East Asia, parts of South America, including the North East of Brazil and also in the Caribbean. Incubation of dengue can be anything between two days to two weeks, averaging around one week. In a majority of cases, there is a sudden onset of symptoms with a high fever and intense, crippling pain in the joints, bones and muscles. The sensation is often one of the bones feeling broken. There can be severe headache and fever which can last for some days. There can be a skin eruption with red patches. In most cases, there is a gradual remission and spontaneous recovery after the intense symptoms have abated but it can take some time. Homeopathy can be important here to help recovery. However, a more serious disease, dengue hemorrhagic fever may occur which can be fatal and needs professional care. There is no effective conventional treatment for dengue fever as it is a viral condition. *See Chapter Six: Common Conditions, Fever and Influenza.*

● HOMEOPATHIC CARE

Aconite, *Belladonna* or *Bryonia* are often needed in the initial stages of the condition where it may seem like any other fever. Each remedy is useful when there is a high fever, which is often dry and burning.

Eupatorium perfoliatum is however the first remedy to think of in dengue is, as it has the characteristic bone breaking pains that are often seen. These pains are felt all over, but especially in the back. There can be an intense headache, fever, chill and often nausea and vomiting. The chill is often felt going up and down the back.

Gelsemium can also look like *Eupatorium*, with aching in the joints and muscles and a chill in the back. However it often has more drowsiness, dullness and weakness and not the pain in the bones so strongly.

Rhus tox also has great aching in the body but with much more restlessness. With the fever, there can be great chill, which is much worse from any uncovering. It can feel as if cold water is being poured over the body.

It may occur that you give one remedy at the beginning of treatment and then need to move to another remedy as the picture changes. One needs to notice the shift in the symptom picture over a number of days. *Aconite* and *Belladonna* may often be indicated at the beginning and the other remedies later. *Bryonia* and *Rhus tox* can often be alternated as the symptom picture changes.

COMBINATION STRATEGY One can combine more than one remedy together, if a clear image is not seen. Choose between the remedies listed. *Eupatorium perfoliatum* however is the most likely remedy to be indicated in this condition.

Malaria

ONSET Symptoms come within 7-14 days of infection.
KEY SYMPTOMS Fever, chill, aching, weakness, sweating. Fever worse at night often, but can feel OK in the day. Periodical fevers, coming every 3-4 days. Great weakness. Diarrhea, which may be the first symptom seen. In children especially great anemia, with swelling of liver and spleen. Complications of meningitis – convulsions, coma, death.

Malaria is the biggest killer of any disease facing the planet, greater than AIDS and TB combined. For a traveler to Africa or parts of Asia, it is the most important disease to protect against. Conventionally, a variety of medications can be taken as a preventative against the disease. Over the years, the recommended medications have changed as the disease has adapted and developed resistance against anti-malaria medications.

For short term travel to very risky parts of the world like Sub Saharan Africa and South East Asia, taking conventional anti-malarials makes sense, but it is important to find one that works for you and to evaluate the risks. Prevention is always the key. For travelers or others who are living in malaria areas for prolonged periods of time (six months or more), taking medication on a long term basis is not so realistic as the longer the medications are taken, the more possible are side effects. However, this is a very individual issue. Some people do fine on them, others do not. There is also a lack of research on the long term effects of anti-malarial medication and so drug companies are not able to make formal recommendations on their use. Also, drugs used to treat malaria can be less effective if medication has been taken for prevention. However, if you do choose to take anti-malarials for more than six months in a row, it is important to find the right drug to take, which is effective, affordable and with minimal side effects. Doxycyclin (an antibiotic) and Mefloquine (Larium) are two of the most common recommended, but each has its side effects, especially if taken for prolonged periods. Also, evaluation of the risks in different areas of a country or countries may allow for a relatively risk free gap in taking medication. However, most 'ex pats' living in tropical areas for prolonged periods do not take anti-malarials as a routine treatment. However, they often have immediate access to appropriate malarial treatment. If you are traveling for prolonged periods in a high risk malaria area and are not going to be near medical care, it is good to take some malaria medication with you in case of an attack. Many long-term 'ex pats' do get bouts of malaria from time to time. Basically, the longer one lives in a malaria country, the more likely one is to get a bout, sooner or later. Over time, most people living in a malarial country do acquire some immunity, depending on general health factors, but once leaving that country, the immunity does not last that long (6 months or so) and on returning, there is an increased risk again. Therefore, it is important to consider what other options there are to both protect and treat malaria. Natural medicines can be used in conjunction with conventional medication or on their own if it seems appropriate.

For shorter trips to malarial countries, the most important issues to consider are evaluating the risks of malaria where you are going and finding the appropriate anti-malarial if you choose to take them. More information on this is given below and much information is available on government and health websites.

Conventional medical channels and government bodies will not recommend most natural treatments, including homeopathy because of the lack of scientific proof that it works. However, in my experience working in Africa and seeing how local homeopaths are able to treat malaria, as well as growing evidence of homeopathy's prophylactic effect, I feel it is useful to have this information and use it, either in conjunction with conventional protocols or on their own if you choose. It is important you do the research and choose a strategy that works for you.

There are two basic forms of malaria. Most common is 'benign malaria' and can show as recurrent intermittent fevers (described often as tertian and quartian malaria) and other associated symptoms. For many living in malarial areas, they may get a new infection once to three times a year, with mild to serious symptoms but which can be treated fairly easily. There will be no attacks in between. The number of infections and seriousness of the attacks depends much on the constitution and basic susceptibility of a person. More serious is 'malignant malaria' in which the liver and spleen can be deeply and quickly affected leading to profound anemia and liver dysfunction. This type of malaria can often be fatal. There is often a lack of the periodicity found in the benign malaria but jaundice, anemia and other serious symptoms are seen in acute phases. Cerebral malaria is one of these conditions and leads to coma, convulsions and possible death. This has to be treated immediately. It is most lethal in young children and those with already weak immune systems. However, in more remote parts of Africa, many people simply have no access to any form of medical care and the largest mortality rates are amongst young malnourished children who cannot access health care of any kind.

Also, for many people in Africa and other endemic countries, there is a form of chronic (benign) malaria, which while not lethal, can generally undermine a person's health. Some people have it worse than others, but it also depends very much on overall immunity and the history of other conditions such as AIDS, T.B., malnutrition, etc. These forms of malaria are quite accessible to natural medicine. Visitors to countries who do get malaria can also experience recurrent bouts of malaria, even after returning to their home country and without subsequent re-infection. This can be treated with the same remedies listed below or with more constitutional homeopathic care.

It is also common for a person living in malaria areas to test positive for malaria yet have no symptoms and then get symptoms when unrelated events occur, such as physical or emotional stress. This can activate the condition as the liver can carry the parasite which then gets released due to stress. Correspondingly, during the first outbreak of symptoms, there can be at times no evidence of infection in blood work. The incubation period can be up to two weeks from infection and the first bout of symptoms often lasts up to one week. The initial fever may last a few hours but after about eight hours, the temperature can be normal. However, within 3 days, another episode can begin (hence the term tertian malaria). Further attacks can occur over weeks until gradually they disappear. However, residual weakness, weight loss and swelling of the spleen and/or liver are quite common. For some people, that will be the end of attacks whereas for others, another bout can occur a few weeks later and after a number of episodes will again disappear until a new episode occurs weeks or months later. A less common type of malaria is called quartian malaria in that attacks occur every 4 days. This form tends to be stronger and more serious than the tertian attacks, with episodes occurring even years later.

There are various strains of malaria, the most dangerous one being Falciparum malaria. This relates to the particular parasitic infection. It is this strain which can cause the cerebral form of malaria that tends to kill young children so easily. It is important to know which type of malaria a person has in order to find the correct conventional treatment. This virulent form is often found in Sub-Saharan Africa, in particular West Africa.

◆ HOMEOPATHIC CARE

Treating malaria can be difficult using traditional homeopathic methodology, especially if one is treating oneself. It is highly recommended to get more professional care if at all possible. As mentioned, homeopathic treatment can be given in conjunction with conventional therapy. The following remedies are the most commonly used homeopathic remedies. The basic care for prevention can also be given at the same time as it is often the same treatment. *(See www.thenaturalmedicineguide.com)*. Also study the main fever and influenza remedies in *Chapter Six: Common Conditions*, as in the acute phase, any remedy may be needed, especially *Aconite*, *Arsenicum album*, *Belladonna*, *Eupatorium perfoliatum*, *Ipecac* and *Nux vomica*.

Acute 1st phase (Benign and Malignant)

At this stage, it may not be clear that it is malaria. It can look like many other diseases, including dengue, influenza, Lassa fever, sunstroke, typhoid etc., and it is important to get tested. However, homeopathic remedies can be given, simply based on the symptom picture. For people who have already had a bout of malaria before, it is more obvious that it is a recurrence. Often there is a relatively sudden onset of fever, with periods of chill, alternating with heat and sweating. There may be extreme shivering in the chill phase. There is often weakness, a lack of appetite and at times diarrhea and vomiting. When experiencing fever or chill, you must stay hydrated. Take oral rehydration as that will help deal with the fever and consequent weakness. Water alone may not be sufficient to replenish fluids.

Arsenicum album is one of the first remedies to consider. There is fever, great shaking chill and a need to be covered. There can be intense nausea, vomiting and at times diarrhea. There is great weakness and restlessness and during the fever often a thirst for sips of water. In this stage the remedy needs to be given frequently, one tsp. every ten to fifteen minutes in water.

Nux vomica is also often indicated and is similar to *Arsenicum album*. There is pain in the abdomen, often with violent intense vomiting and urging for stool. There can be pains in the liver and spleen which is much worse from any touch to the region. *Belladonna* is needed when sudden, intense, very hot and dry fever is seen.

Eupatorium perfoliatum is a good remedy when there are intense aching pains in the bones, feeling as if they would break. This is throughout the body, including the back. There can be great nausea and vomiting, often of bile and great, shaking chill.

Ipecac has intense nausea and vomiting in all stages, along with a fever. There can be a great sinking feeling in the stomach. There may be no thirst, even in heat, but often can have a clean tongue.

China may also be needed in the acute stage when there is a marked periodicity to symptoms but more often is indicated when there is an ongoing recurrence of symptoms or in particularly intense bouts of malaria when the liver and spleen are swollen. *See malignant malaria below and Chapter Six: Common Conditions, Fever section.*

COMBINATION STRATEGY If the picture is not clear, put one tablet of all the remedies above in a glass and take a sip (one tsp.) every ten to fifteen minutes for four hours and then once hourly after this. Look for some relief in four hours to one day but it will take longer to see serious improvement. As mentioned, it is hard to find the exact remedy so combining all the remedies ensures that ideally one of them will work.

Chronic recurrence (Benign)

China is needed when there is a fever that comes in exact phases and there can be great ringing in the ears. There is great fatigue and often abdominal fullness and pain and swelling in the liver area. In the fever stage, there can be drenching sweats which are exhausting. There can be great abdominal bloating, a lack of appetite and diarrhea. (Also to be considered are *Chinium arsenicosum* – when nausea and vomiting and extreme weakness are felt and *Chinium sulphuricum* – when dizziness and tinnitus predominate and also exact periodicity of complaints).

Natrum muriaticum is given in more chronic conditions when there is an intense, splitting headache, weakness, perspiration, great thirst and fever that comes in marked phases. *Sulphur* needs to be given if other remedies have been given and do not work fully and you feel just exhausted and flat, but without any other clear symptoms.

Baptisia and *Pyrogen* can also be given when the malaria fever has become totally exhausting and you feel simply exhausted and prostrated, with fever and aching, and a bruised soreness over the whole body. *See Chapter Six: Common Conditions, Influenza section.*

NOTE These remedies can also be indicated in the acute first phase and especially *China* can be combined with other remedies in the first phases of malaria. Even if you are taking conventional medication for malaria, you can still take some homeopathic remedies to help. Or after finishing medication you can see what symptoms are remaining and give a remedy. If in doubt, simply take *China* 30c, twice daily for one week to aid recovery.

Malignant Malaria

Often the liver and spleen are affected (and also with benign malaria), and profound anemia is seen. This needs to be treated by a medical expert and conventional therapy given. Homeopathic remedies can be used alongside as necessary. *Ceanothus* is a specific remedy for swelling of the liver and spleen with anemia. It should ideally be given in a low potency, e.g., 6c and repeated frequently for one to two weeks. *China* has swelling of the liver and of the whole abdomen. There is jaundice and anemia with great bloating and little appetite. There is great weakness. *Chinium arsenicosum* is also a useful remedy when there is profound weakness, anemia, nausea and vomiting. These remedies can be given in a 6c or 30c potency and repeated 3 times daily for at least one week.

🌿 HERBAL CARE

These are more effective in the acute and chronic relapse phases. Neem tincture (Azadrachita indica – Margosa bark), Artemisia annua (Sweet wormwood), Eucalyptus (in a tincture from the leaves and/or in a homeopathic potency up to 6x or 6c).

These should be given up to ten times a day in tincture, five drops each time. They can be taken along with homeopathic remedies. Neem and artemesia can also be taken in a tea form (5-10 grams of dried leaf, 1tr of boiling water poured over them and drunk slowly through the day. Make separately. Use less for children. 10 grams is used in more serious cases. Pregnant women should not use this, especially in first trimester). Knowing a good source of neem and artemisia is useful and both are widely found in the tropics. Lemon grass tea should be taken for any fever, 1-2 liters daily.

Typhoid

ONSET Incubation is between 7-10 days. Easily confused with malaria in early stages and also yellow fever (see end of chapter)

KEY SYMPTOMS Fever resembling influenza, sore throat, abdominal pains. Fever coming and going. High fever in children with diarrhea, vomiting. After 1-2 weeks, diarrhea becomes worse, great weakness, fever becomes more debilitating with weakness and delirium. Lung symptoms with bloody mucus with cough. Bloody stools, leading to perforation of the bowels.

Typhoid is a bacterial infection and is one of the most serious and common conditions in the tropical regions of the world. For travelers, the Indian subcontinent, Sub Saharan Africa and Latin America carry the most risk. It is caught from food or water contaminated with Salmonella bacteria. The incubation period for typhoid is around ten days, but can be less than that, as well as much longer (which should be considered if one gets sick even weeks after returning home). Even though there are characteristic symptoms of the disease as it develops, in many cases the disease can go unnoticed until serious symptoms develop. Often it looks similar to influenza, with a general unwell feeling, fever, sore throat, cough and generalized abdominal pains. One of the most characteristic qualities about typhoid is that the pulse can remain unusually low even though the temperature is rising. This is one of the most important things to notice if typhoid is suspected. However, in many cases, this may not be seen but typhoid always needs to be considered in such situations and a test can be done, especially to differentiate from malaria as it is not uncommon to see a fever come and go in apparent phases. (At this point the homeopathic remedy may not be obvious but pay careful attention to the symptoms). Symptoms in children may be serious, with high fever, diarrhea and vomiting and also with a stiff neck, resembling meningitis. There may even be convulsions.

At the beginning, there may simply be some loose stools. Then after one to two weeks, a fever begins and there can be constipation at this point, and often a generalized body pain and headache. As the symptoms develop into the second week there are more distinct abdominal symptoms with sensitivity around the appendix area and the liver and spleen become swollen. Symptoms can get worse into the third week, with diarrhea developing and great weakness, confusion, disorientation and even delirium. There can be a severe headache, especially felt in the neck area. If untreated, this can last weeks, with symptoms changing but no real recovery. There can be intestinal bleeding even leading to perforation of the bowel. Other complications of typhoid include pneumonia, inflammation of the heart, acute arthritis, abscess of the spleen and other conditions. Gradually recovery will take place if there are not serious complications.

Because of the difficulty in diagnosis, it is important that treatment is begun as soon as possible. Conventional treatment can be effective in these cases, including the need for blood transfusions, and rehydration. However, homeopathic treatment can also be given alongside any conventional treatment and can greatly help the body recover from this disease. The earlier homeopathic and conventional treatment is given, the better the prognosis. However, a clear picture for a homeopathic remedy is not always obvious in the beginning. Try and wait until the picture becomes clear.

Even after recovery, some people still excrete the typhoid bacteria in the feces and urine for a number of months. Therefore, these people can spread the disease unbeknownst to themselves and others. It is also important that the patient is well looked after during the period of recovery, with simple, clean food, juices and water. Heavy food, dairy and meat should be avoided. Recovery can be quite slow. *See Chapter Five: Digestive Conditions, Diarrhea and Dysentery; Chapter Six: Common Conditions, Fever and Influenza.*

◆ HOMEOPATHIC CARE

Most important remedies needed are described in Chapter Six. One can give homeopathic remedies even when conventional treatment is given.

Arsenicum album is often indicated in the beginning stages, and the most important symptoms are weakness, chill, restlessness and anxiety.

Rhus tox is indicated when there is great aching and restlessness. There is often a great chill and desire to be covered and the body feels as if dashed with water. There is a chill in single parts of the body. The aching is intense, with rheumatic type symptoms, which can be stitching, tearing and shooting, with great restlessness.

Baptisia is the first remedy to consider once it is in the second stage of the condition. There is great prostration, with weakness and aching of muscles. One can't get comfortable, and the bed feels hard.

There is a dullness and confusion in the mind. Parts of the body feel scattered over the bed or feels is in pieces. One falls asleep when answering questions in a passive type of delirium. The face often looks dusky, besotted and stupid. Fever is low but it's as if one sinks into the bed and there is an offensive odor from the body.

Bryonia and *Gelsemium* have to be compared with *Baptisia*, in both the first and second stage of typhoid. *Bryonia* has symptoms of a fever with delirium. One wants to be quiet and be left alone. In a delirium, one can say "I want to go home", even though there. Pains are worse from any motion or jar. There is often a great headache, as if the head is splitting open and is much worse from any motion or coughing. Joints can be inflamed and swollen and there is soreness in the abdomen, which is worse from pressure.

Gelsemium has symptoms of weakness, heaviness, soreness and sleepiness. Eyelids look very heavy and the face sleepy. There is a low state of fever with a severe headache, especially in the back of the head, (occipital). Mentally, there is dullness, confusion and often dizziness. With fever, there is often chill, with great aching and chill is found going up and down the back. Often there is a lack of thirst during the heat phase of fever.

Ipecac is indicated when there is great nausea and respiratory symptoms with cough and bleeding from the lungs. There can be a profuse nose bleeding with cough and other symptoms. The cough is suffocating and there is rattling in the chest without expectoration. It is indicated more in the second stage of typhoid.

Phosphorus also has similar respiratory symptoms with coughing and bleeding from the lungs and with nosebleed. The cough is often hacking and dry, with a great tightness around the chest. Ideally at this stage you will have professional medical help.

Muriatic acidum is indicated in more serious typhoid cases, with great prostration and aching of muscles. Mucous membranes of the mouth are dry, bleeding, cracked and ulcerated and the face is dark red. There is great soreness of the body causing restlessness. There is muttering with loud moaning and there can be intense burning heat with aversion to covers. It will often be compared with *Baptisia* and also *Pyrogen*.

Pyrogen is indicated in the second stage, when the fever becomes 'septic', and one feels an intense, bruised soreness, with bone pains and the odor of the body and breath is foul. The pulse is either very quick or very slow. With a fever, there can be excitability, loquacity or great confusion, and like with *Baptisia*, a sense of duality in the body. Chills are often felt between the shoulder blades. It is given when other remedies have not worked well and you are sinking lower into the disease. Hopefully medical help will be available in such circumstances.

COMBINATION STRATEGY Given the complexity of the disease and the difficulty finding the correct homeopathic remedy, one can mix together a number of remedies to cover the situation. However, if a picture is clear, then give the single remedy first. This is the best way to approach this. But if necessary, mix together *Arsenicum album*, *Baptisia*, *Bryonia*, *Gelsemium* and *Rhus tox* if aching and low mental states are dominant, even with delirium. If hemorrhage is seen, then mix together *Ipecac* and *Phosphorus*. If low, septic states predominate, mix together **Baptisia**, **Muriatic acid** and **Pyrogen**. Improvement may be slow but some signs should be seen in one to two days. The remedy should be repeated in water, one tsp. every one to two hours when it is severe and only reduced when symptoms improve. It should still be given two to three times a day for at least one week.

If a single remedy is given and the picture changes stop the remedy and consider a new remedy. Do not wait too long. Another remedy should be found if there is a change of symptoms. However, if a remedy is working, do not change it. Continue until a new picture emerges. In typhoid, recovery is slow, even with the correct remedy.

Yellow fever is a viral infection from mosquito bites. As mentioned it is rarely seen for travelers and there is a mandatory vaccine for travel in endemic areas. The vaccine should be avoided though when there is an egg allergy and for people with immune problems. Ensure you get an examption certificate from your doctor. Remedies indicated include most of the malaria and typhoid remedies, especially **Arsenicum album**, **Nux vomica** and **China**. **Lachesis** is also indicated if spontaneous bruising and bleeding is seen.

⬤ HERBAL CARE

Take eucalyptus tincture – and/or homeopathic dose of 6x or 6c. It should be taken three to four times a day at the beginning of any symptoms. **Echinacea** tincture can also be taken.

Chapter Nine
Remedy List

The following 52 remedies are some of the most essential remedies used for travel situations and general home care and which are found in most homeopathic kits. Some other remedies are mentioned in the manual but not listed here, but which are included in the larger travel guide, *The Natural Medicine Guide for Travel and Home*. If traveling in more remote places or where homeopathic and herbal remedies may not be found, then the most important remedies should be carried with you including some remedies not normally found in kits.

For a complete list of information on remedies mentioned in the book go to **www.thenaturalmedicineguide.com**.

Homeopathic Remedies

ACONITE monkshood

CONDITIONS Accidents and Injury, Anxiety, Bites, Burns, Colds, Coughs, Dengue fever, Ear pain, Emergencies and

Disasters, Fainting, Fever, Fright,, Influenza, Malaria, Poisoning, Shock.

KEY SYMPTOMS Sudden, intense and extreme symptoms. Fever high, burning, dry and sweaty, with great restlessness and thirst. Great anxiety and anguish, terror. Ailments from anxiety, fright, shock.

COMPARE Belladonna, Chamomilla, Coffea, Gelsemium.

ALLIUM CEPA onion

CONDITIONS Allergies, Colds, Conjunctivitis, Coughs.

KEY SYMPTOMS Streaming, burning eyes, nose runs profusely, with sneezing. Dry, tearing cough from larynx, with hoarseness. Pains like needles, shooting along the lines of nerves.

COMPARE Euphrasia, Sabadilla.

ALOE socotrine aloes

CONDITIONS Diarrhea.

KEY SYMPTOMS Great insecurity in the bowel, cannot pass wind without losing stool. Emotionally a feeling of insecurity, being in unfamiliar places, not having control of situation. Stools with mucus jelly and loud flatus, sputtering and/or hot, involuntary. Pain in the back.

COMPARE Arsenicum album, Podophyllum, Sulphur.

ANTIMONIUM TARTARICUM tartar emetic

CONDITIONS Bilharzia, Coughs (bronchitis, pneumonia), Influenza.

KEY SYMPTOMS Indicated for more serious infections. Cough deep, loose, suffocating. Feels as if drowning. Fluid in lungs, respiration rattling and wheezing but little mucus raised and difficult breathing with cough. Face pale and sweating. Lungs feeling paralyzed.

COMPARE Arsenicum album, Ipecac.

APIS honey bee

CONDITIONS Allergies, Bites, Cystitis (Kidney), Fever, Hives

KEY SYMPTOMS Affected area is red, swollen, puffy or hard swelling. Intense stinging, burning pains worse from warmth and better cold. Feeling of irritation, both physically and emotionally. Allergic reaction to any bite, sting. Inflammations of skin and organs with burning, stinging pains. No thirst during heat. In kidneys, pain is bursting, with fullness in bladder and burning urine.

COMPARE Arsenicum album, Cantharis, Ledum, Rhus tox, Urtica urens.

ARNICA leopard's bane

CONDITIONS Accidents and Injuries, Altitude sickness, Appendicitis, Burns, Concussion, Emergencies and Disasters,

Eye Conditions, Fractures, Hemorrhage, Injuries, Jetlag, Pain, Shock, Spinal injury, Sprains, Wounds.

KEY SYMPTOMS First remedy for all injuries and shock. Bruised, soreness of injured part. Head injuries, including concussion. For states of shock, says he is fine when not. After effects of any exertion – stiffness, sore, bruised. Fever, when feeling sore and bruised and the bed feels hard.

COMPARE Aconite, Baptisia, Hypericum, Ledum, Natrum sulph, Rhus tox.

ARSENICUM ALBUM white oxide of arsenic

CONDITIONS Allergies, Asthma, Bites, Burns, Cholera, Colds, Coughs, Diarrhea, Dysentery, Emergencies and Disasters, Fever, Food poisoning, Hiccough, Indigestion, Influenza, Malaria, Nausea, Poison oak, Poisoning, Typhoid, Ulcers, Yellow fever.

KEY SYMPTOMS Restlessness and anxiety. Anguish and fear. Great weakness. Burning pains and discharges. Diarrhea watery, profuse, offensive. All infections of stomach and abdomen. Great nausea and vomiting and profuse watery, burning diarrhea. Acute asthma with great anxiety. Fever, with restlessness, anxiety and great chill. May have internal burning. Easily exhausted. High fever, sweats, thirst for small sips.

COMPARE Aconite, Camphor, Carbo veg, China, Rhus tox, Veratrum album.

BAPTISIA wild indigo

CONDITIONS Dysentery, Influenza, Malaria, Typhoid.
KEY SYMPTOMS Serious infectious conditions, great soreness,
exhaustion and depletion. Stools dark, thin, bloody, very
offensive. Distension and rumbling. Low mental state, tiredness,
confusion, falls asleep easily, even when spoken to. Face is
besotted and dark red. Ongoing 'septic' low fever.
COMPARE Arnica, Arsenicum album, Bryonia, Eupatorium
perf, Gelsemium, Muriatic acid, Pyrogen, Rhus tox.

BELLADONNA deadly nightshade

CONDITIONS Appendicitis, Bites, Boils, Breast issues,
Conjunctivitis, Coughs, Cystitis, Dengue fever, Diaper rash,
Ear pain, Fever, German measles, Heatstroke, Hemorrhage,
Influenza, Kidney, Malaria, Measles, Rabies, Sinusitis,
Teething, Throat Conditions.
KEY SYMPTOMS Sudden and intense conditions. Pains bursting,
sharp, throbbing. High burning fevers, thirst for sips, lemonade.
Jarring aggravates. Wild mental state with fever, pupils dilated.
Delirium. Aggression in fever. Redness of affected part, great heat.
Cough hard, intense, violent.
COMPARE Aconite, Apis, Bryonia, Drosera, Glonoinum,
Stramonium, Sulphur.

BRYONIA wild hops

CONDITIONS Accidents and Injuries, Appendicitis, Breast issues, Colds, Colic, Constipation, Coughs, Dengue fever, Fever, Fractures, Influenza, Injuries, Pain, Sprains, Typhoid.
KEY SYMPTOMS All motion aggravates, desire to keep totally still. Holds chest or head when coughing. Cough hard, dry, painful. Easily irritated, wants to be left alone. Slowly developing inflammation and fever. Dryness, especially mouth and mucous membranes. Great thirst. Delirium, saying "they want to go home", although there. Achiness, motion aggravates and worse from any jar. Injury to joints and bones with excruciating pain, worse motion.
COMPARE Baptisia, Belladonna, Gelsemium, Rhus tox.

CALENDULA marigold

CONDITIONS Wounds.
KEY SYMPTOMS Antiseptic and healing for wounds, especially cuts, lacerations and punctured wounds. Applied locally in tincture and creams. Given internally when wounds are painful with cutting pains.
COMPARE Hypericum, Ledum, Staphysagria.

CANTHARIS spanish fly

CONDITIONS Burns, Cystitis, Kidney.
KEY SYMPTOMS Constant, violent urge to urinate, only a few

drops being passed. Burning and cutting pains with urination.
Great intensity of symptoms, cannot stand pain and urging.
Blood in the urine. Second and third degree burns, extreme
burning, blisters and oozing of moisture. Extreme pain, feelings
of anguish and frenzy.

COMPARE Apis, Belladonna, Berberis, Causticum, Sarsaparilla,
Urtica urens.

CARBO VEG vegetable charcoal

CONDITIONS Coughs (pneumonia), Emergencies and
Disasters, Fainting, Indigestion, Influenza, Poisoning, Shock,
Ulcers, Yellow Fever.

KEY SYMPTOMS Weakness and collapsed states. Ailments from
shock, exhaustion. Coldness and yet a craving for air. Wants
to be fanned. Looks like death. Lacks oxygen, turning blue.
Exhausted state of any disease, much weakness, breathlessness.
Great distension of abdomen. Loud and rancid burping and
farting, all food turns to gas. Clothing around waist aggravates.
Worse from ice cream, fruit and rich food.

COMPARE Camphor, China, Veratrum album.

CHAMOMILLA chamomille

CONDITIONS Anger, Colic, Diaper rash, Diarrhea, Ear pain,
Menstrual issues, Pain, Pregnancy and Birth, Sleeplessness,
Spinal injury, Teething, Toothache.

KEY SYMPTOMS Extreme reaction to very small things. Great impatience, irritability and anger, nothing will satisfy. Capriciousness. Pain out of proportion to situation. Children cannot be satisfied, shriek all the time, as if in agony. Colic, teething and diarrhea of children. Stools green, like grass, slimy, with food in, smelling of bad eggs.

COMPARE Aconite, Belladonna, Borax, Cina, Nux vomica.

CHINA quinine

CONDITIONS Diarrhea, Dysentery, Hemorrhage, Hepatitis, Malaria, Typhoid, Yellow Fever.

KEY SYMPTOMS Weakness and exhaustion, after diarrhea, fever, stool and loss of fluids. First remedy for Giardiasis. Fullness in the abdomen and stomach. Very little appetite. Easily full after few mouthfuls. Fullness, hardness and pains in abdomen and liver. Swelling of liver and spleen. Much gas, no relief from passing. Hepatitis. Bloody, mucus stool, of undigested food. Diarrhea alternating with constipation. Diarrhea worse fruit and rich food. Periodical fevers, with chill, malarial fever.

COMPARE Arsenicum album, Carbo veg, Chelidonium, Natrum muriaticum, Nux vomica, Sulphur.

COCCULUS indian cockle

CONDITIONS Concussion, Fainting, Fright, Grief, Jet lag, Nausea, Sleeplessness, Spinal Injury, Travel sickness.

KEY SYMPTOMS Problems from lack of sleep and anxiety and worry. Weakness and exhaustion from worry. Dizziness, heaviness in body, especially head. Travel sickness, with nausea, vomiting and great dizziness. Has to lie down, worse on sitting, rising. Ailments from grief, fright, shock and loss of sleep.
COMPARE Gelsemium, Ignatia, Tabacum.

COFFEA CRUDA coffee

CONDITIONS Anxiety, Sleeplessness, Toothache.
KEY SYMPTOMS Great over-excitability, nervousness, irritability and anxiety. Sleeplessness from too many thoughts, excitability. Over-sensitivity to everything, to noises, smells etc. Constantly feeling on edge. Great sensitivity to pain, especially teeth, worse touch and noise, better with ice. Weeping with pain.
COMPARE Chamomilla, Colocynthis, Nux vomica, Staphysagria.

COLOCYNTHIS bitter cucumber

CONDITIONS Anger, Colic, Diarrhea, Indigestion, Menstrual issues, Pain.
KEY SYMPTOMS Violent, intense cramping, cutting and twisting pains in the abdomen, has to bend double and/or press hands into abdomen. Restlessness with the pain, twisting and turning. Ailments from anger, indignation. Suppression of emotions.
COMPARE Magnesium phosphoricum, Nux vomica, Staphysagria.

DROSERA sundew

CONDITIONS Coughs, Whooping cough.

KEY SYMPTOMS Cough is racking, barking, painful spasmodic, violent. First remedy in whooping cough, croup. Retching and vomiting, red or blue face with cough. Painful cough, holds chest. Cough worse lying down, laughing and talking. Hoarse voice with cough.

COMPARE Aconite, Belladonna, Bryonia, Coccus cacti, Cuprum, Hepar sulph, Ipecac, Spongia

ECHINACEA echinacea

CONDITIONS Bites, Wounds.

KEY SYMPTOMS Wounds that are infected and gangrenous.

COMPARE Arnica, Lachesis.

EUPATORIUM PERFOLIATUM boneset

CONDITIONS Dengue fever, Fever, Fractures, Influenza, Malaria.

KEY SYMPTOMS Intense aching and pain in bones as if breaking and bruised. Aching in the back. Violent shaking chill, felt worse in back, moving up and down. Nausea and bitter vomiting, of bile. Increased thirst. Intense headache. Nausea, worse smell of food.

COMPARE Arnica, Arsenicum album, Baptisia, Gelsemium, Nux vomica, Rhus tox.

EUPHRASIA eyebright

CONDITIONS Allergies, Conjunctivitis, Whooping cough.

KEY SYMPTOMS Eyes are burning, watery and red. Simple conjunctivitis. Irritation in eyes from profuse watery discharge. Yellow/green discharge from eyes. Whooping cough with profuse lachrymation and watery nasal discharge.

COMPARE Allium cepa, Drosera, Pulsatilla.

GELSEMIUM yellow jasmine

CONDITIONS Anxiety, Concussion, Dengue fever, Diarrhea, Fainting, Fever, Fright, Heatstroke, Influenza, Pregnancy and Birth, Shock, Spinal injury, Typhoid.

KEY SYMPTOMS Fever with great aching and heaviness of the body, especially in muscles and back. Drowsy, weak, dizzy, confused and often thirst less. Fever develops slowly. Great chills, especially going up and down the back. Eyelids are heavy, and face is besotted. The head is heavy and needs support. Anticipatory anxiety, with diarrhea, trembling. Ailments from fright, grief, shock.

COMPARE Aconite, Baptisia, Bryonia, Cocculus, Eupatorium perfoliatum, Ignatia.

HEPAR SULPH calcium sulphide (Hahnemann)

CONDITIONS Boils, Coughs, Ear pain, Throat Conditions.

KEY SYMPTOMS Infections with stitching, sharp pains as if a needle inserted. Sensation of splinter, especially in ear, throat, chest and skin. Pains in ear shooting to throat and vice versa, worse swallowing and coughing. Worse cold, wind and better warmth. Offensive discharge from ears. Boils and abscesses have sharp, stitching pains, worse touch and cold air. Suppurating wounds, splinters. Anger and extreme touchiness. Cough dry, intense, barking and painful. Also loose, with great rattling and hoarseness.

COMPARE Aconite, Drosera, Mercurius, Nux vomica, Silicea, Spongia.

HYPERICUM St. Johns wort

CONDITIONS Accidents and Injuries, Concussion, Pain, Spinal injury, Wounds.

KEY SYMPTOMS Injuries to nerve rich areas, with sharp, intense, shooting pains. Pain unendurable. Crushed finger tips, lacerated wounds which are very painful. Head injuries, especially to occiput, spinal nerves.

COMPARE Arnica, Ledum.

IGNATIA St. Ignatius bean

CONDITIONS Fainting, Grief, Hiccough, Shock, Sleeplessness.

KEY SYMPTOMS Sudden shock, disappointment and sadness. First remedy in acute grief. Choking in the throat, difficult to swallow and difficult to breathe, often with sighing breath.

Violent weeping or can't weep at all.

COMPARE Aconite, Gelsemium, Natrum mur, Nux vomica, Pulsatilla.

IPECAC ipecac

CONDITIONS Bilharzia, Bronchitis, Coughs, Emergencies and Disasters, Hemorrhage, Influenza, Malaria, Nausea, Teething, Typhoid, Whooping cough.

KEY SYMPTOMS Nausea with all complaints especially with bleeding. Cough is intense, violent, incessant and racking. Loose, coarse rattle in the chest yet little mucus is raised. Face is red with the intensity of cough with gagging and retching. Whooping cough, asthma.

COMPARE Antimonium tart, Coccus cacti, Drosera, Hepar sulph.

LACHESIS surucucu snake poison

CONDITIONS Boils, Bites, Bronchitis, Coughs (pneumonia), Diphtheria, Frostbite, Influenza, Menstrual issues, Menopause, Throat Conditions, Ulcers, Yellow fever.

KEY SYMPTOMS Infection of left side of throat, pain worse swallowing air or liquid more than food. Lump in throat, choking feeling. Dislike of clothing, pressure on throat. Cold drinks relieve and warm drinks aggravate. Serious bites and infections on skin when purple, swollen and looks infected,

turning blue/black. Snake and spider bites. Serious pneumonia with hemorrhage from lungs and skin is purplish/blue.
COMPARE Apis, Crotalus horridus, Ledum, Pyrogen, Tarentula cubensis.

LEDUM marsh tea

CONDITIONS Accidents and Injuries, Bites, Eye Conditions-injuries, Injuries, Lyme disease, Sprains, Tetanus, Wounds.
KEY SYMPTOMS First remedy for most bites and stings. Punctured wounds. Tetanus prevention. Swelling, puffiness, redness of injured part. Can feel cold to the touch. Injuries to joints and muscles and eyes. Bruising and swelling around eye. Injuries to joints with swelling, better cold applications. Prevention of Lyme disease and for joint pains after tick bites.
COMPARE Apis, Arnica, Hypericum.

LYCOPODIUM club moss

CONDITIONS Colic, Bladder, Hepatitis.
KEY SYMPTOMS For bladder and kidney conditions, especially right kidney with acute colic and kidney stones. Pains extending from right kidney to bladder. Red sand in urine, great pain passing urine. Bloating of abdomen with pains, passing of gas and aversion of clothing around the waist and back. Hepatitis, liver swollen and painful, pain extending to back and right shoulder, with fullness in abdomen, appetite less or increased,

but full after few mouthfuls.
COMPARE Berberis, Chelidonium, China, Sarsaparilla.

MAGNESIUM PHOSPHORICUM phosphate of magnesia

CONDITIONS Colic, Pain, Teething, Toothache.
KEY SYMPTOMS Cramping, spasms in abdomen, forcing to
bend double and better from great pressure and heat. Bloating
in abdomen, loosens clothing, much flatus passed.
COMPARE Coffea, Colocynthis.

MERCURIUS mercury

CONDITIONS Boils, Dysentery, Ear pain, Fungal infections,
Hemorrhage, Hepatitis, Mouth ulcers, Throat Conditions,
Toothache, Ulcers.
KEY SYMPTOMS Offensive taste in the mouth, or metallic taste
with much salivation. Easy sweating, often offensive, and a weak
depleted state. Skin looks dirty. Frequent, painful urging for
bloody very offensive stool with no relief after stool. Weakness
after stool. Ulcerative conditions, ulcers and canker sores in the
mouth. Indicated in more serious and chronic states. Fullness
in the liver region. Hepatitis. Throat infections, with swollen
lymph glands, pains moving from throat to ear and back again.
COMPARE China, Hepar sulph, Mercurius corrosivus, Sulphur.

NATRUM MURIATICUM salt

CONDITIONS Cold sores, Grief, Malaria, Pregnancy and Birth.
KEY SYMPTOMS Great sadness and grief but unable to cry,
stillness of emotions. Everything feels held in, suppressed. In fevers
(malarial) coming exactly the same time each day or every two to
seven days. Fever with great pounding, throbbing headache, as if
hammers in head. Headache from sun. Cold sores from sun.
COMPARE China, Ignatia.

NATRUM SULPHURICUM glaubers salt – sulphate of soda

CONDITIONS Concussion, Spinal injury.
KEY SYMPTOMS Chronic affects of head injury. Headaches,
depression and confusion. Any condition in which a head
injury initiated events.
COMPARE Arnica.

NUX VOMICA poison nut

CONDITIONS Allergies, Anger, Colds, Colic, Constipation,
Cystitis (kidney), Diarrhea, Emergency and Disasters, Fever,
Food poisoning, Hangover, Hemorrhoids, Hepatitis, Hiccough,
Indigestion, Jetlag, Malaria, Menstrual issues, Nausea, Sleep-
lessness, Spinal injury, Toothache, Travel sickness, Yellow fever.
KEY SYMPTOMS Irritation, impatience and frustration with
many complaints. Intense, spasmodic and stitching pains,
especially digestive area. Violent nausea, retching and vomiting.

Ineffectual desire to vomit or pass stool, great urging but no stool. Ailments from too much rich food, stimulants, alcohol. Hangover. Headache with great sensitivity to noise and smells. Insomnia from too much stimulants or too much worry and excitement. Violent shaking chill, must be covered.

COMPARE Arsenicum album, Coffea, Colocynthis, Hepar sulph, Rhus tox, Sulphur.

OPIUM opium

CONDITIONS Fright, Shock.

KEY SYMPTOMS Ailments from intense fright, e.g., seeing accidents, being in war situations. Fear remains, numbness of feelings, easily startled.

COMPARE Aconite, Gelsemium, Stramonium.

PHOSPHORUS phosphorus

CONDITIONS Coughs (Bronchitis, Pneumonia), Emergency and Disasters, Hemorrhage, Hepatitis, Influenza, Typhoid.

KEY SYMPTOMS Intense, hacking, tickling cough with any chest infection, Great tightness in the chest with the cough. Empty, hollow feeling in chest. Hemorrhage, of lungs, bloody expectoration with cough. Bronchitis and pneumonia. Either lobe affected. Easily losing weight with sickness. Easy nose-bleeds. Uterine hemorrhage with bright blood.

COMPARE Drosera, Ipecac, Spongia.

PHYTOLACCA pokeroot

CONDITIONS Breast issues, Throat Conditions.

KEY SYMPTOMS Breasts feel hard and inflamed, with nodular enlargement, even to the armpits. Ulceration/abscess of breasts, of nursing mothers. Nipples are cracked and breast milk is deficient. For inflammation of throat, with stiffness of neck, swelling of tonsils and lymph glands. Pains worse from warm drinks and better from cool.

COMPARE Bryonia, Hepar sulph, Mercurius, Silicea.

PODOPHYLLUM may apple

CONDITIONS Diarrhea, Food poisoning.

KEY SYMPTOMS Much rumbling, gurgling and bloating in the abdomen, and also cramping, which is worse before stool. Stool explosive and forceful. Involuntary stool, even in sleep. Fullness in liver area.

COMPARE Aloe, Sulphur, Veratrum album.

PULSATILLA wind flower

CONDITIONS Breast issues, Chicken pox, Conjunctivitis, Coughs, Ear pain, Grief, Indigestion, Menses, Pregnancy, Styes.

KEY SYMPTOMS Emotional, great weepiness, sadness and clinginess. Children who need extra attention all the time. Demanding. Yellow/green discharge from the eyes, ears or nose. Ear pain worse in a warm room, and feels better in open air.

Everything better in the open air. Sadness, grief, feeling all alone.
COMPARE Euphrasia, Ignatia.

RHUS TOX poison oak (Rhus diversoloba)

CONDITIONS Accident and Injuries, Allergies, Chicken pox,
Cold sores, Dengue fever, Diaper rash, Impetigo, Influenza,
Injuries, Poison oak, Spinal injury, Sprains, Shingles, Typhoid.
KEY SYMPTOMS Injuries to muscles, tendons and joints.
Stiffness and pain, worse on initial motion and better from
continued walking, until tired. Relief from warm applications
and worse from the cold. In fevers, great achiness and rest-
lessness. Tossing and turning at night, with pain and anxiety.
Great chill, has to be covered, averse any uncovering. Any fever
with great chill, aching and restlessness.
COMPARE Arsenicum album, Baptisia, Bryonia, Eupatorium
perf, Gelsemium, Nux vomica.

RUTA GRAV rue

CONDITIONS Accidents and Injuries, Eye Conditions-injuries,
Spinal injury.
KEY SYMPTOMS Injuries to muscles, tendons, ligaments,
periosteum and bones. Symptoms similar to Rhus tox, with sore,
bruised stiffness, better from walking. Injuries to smaller joints,
elbows, knees, wrists and ankles. Tennis elbow, simple eyestrain.
COMPARE Rhus tox, Symphytum.

SARSAPARILLA sarsaparilla

CONDITIONS Cystitis, Kidney.

KEY SYMPTOMS Important remedy to consider in cystitis and kidney infections. Burning pain at the end of urination. Chill in the urethra spreading up to the bladder. Gas passes from the bladder. Women may need to stand to urinate.

COMPARE Cantharis.

SEPIA inky juice of cuttlefish

CONDITIONS   Menstrual issues and Menopause, Nausea, Poisoning, Pregnancy

KEY SYMPTOMS Nausea with great aversion to smell, taste of food. Nausea from poisoning, in pregnancy. Miscarriage and labor issues. Great bearing down feeling in uterus better sitting. Emotionally flat and indifferent to having child.

COMPARE Arsenicum album, Lactic acid, Sabina.

SILICEA pure flint

CONDITIONS Boils, Eye Conditions-chalazion, Teething, Toothache, Worms, Wounds.

KEY SYMPTOMS For children, who have worms with itching and are losing weight with no appetite. Become more reserved and timid and avoid company due to lack of confidence. Chilly and have profuse, sour perspiration. For splintered wounds, especially when beginning to fester. Sharp, splintered pains.

Helps expel splinters and other 'foreign' objects. Mothers whose milk is not tolerated by child. Breasts are hard and inflamed.
COMPARE Calcarea carbonica, Cina, Hepar sulph, Sabadilla.

STAPHYSAGRIA stavesacre

CONDITIONS Anger, Animals(bites), Cystitis, Eye Conditions-Blepharitis, Styes, Wounds.
KEY SYMPTOMS Cystitis which begins after sex – 'Honeymoon Cystitis'. Anger with suppressed emotions, indignation and humiliation. Any physical or emotional feeling of violation. Wounds, especially lacerations to vulnerable areas, e.g., genitalia.
COMPARE Colocynthis, Calendula, Cantharis, Hypericum, Sarsaparilla.

STRAMONIUM datura, thorn apple

CONDITIONS Emergencies and Disasters, Fever, Fright, Rabies, Shock.
KEY SYMPTOMS Ailments from extreme fright, violence. Terror remains after fright. For suspected rabies or intense fever, with symptoms of intense rage, wild delirium, cursing and violent behavior. Extreme violence with unusual strength and mania. Extreme fear and terror, especially of dark, dogs and being alone. Profound aversion to and fear of water, glistening objects and reflections. Aversion to drinking water, with spasms of throat. Brain inflammations (meningitis and encephalitis) with above symptoms.

COMPARE Agaricus, Belladonna, Lyssin, Opium.

SULPHUR sulphur

CONDITIONS Bronchitis, Chicken pox, Conjunctivitis, Coughs, Diarrhea, Dysentery, Ear pain, Fever, Hemorrhoids, Indigestion, Scabies, Worms.

KEY SYMPTOMS When other remedies have only partially worked, some fever or other symptoms remain and they feel simply not right, lacking energy and interest. Great burning and heat in affected area. Offensive hot diarrhea, like sulphur. Urging for stool at 5am, or on waking. Great hunger and weakness at 11am. Mentally low spirited and indifferent. Skin looks dirty.

COMPARE Arsenicum album, Mercurius, Nux vomica.

SYMPHYTUM comfrey

CONDITIONS Accidents and Injuries, Fractures, Eye Conditions-Injuries.

KEY SYMPTOMS Injuries to bones, especially facial bones. Follows Arnica and Ledum when cheekbone is damaged or broken. Heals bones and given after broken bone has been set.

COMPARE Arnica, Ledum, Rhus tox.

TABACUM tobacco

CONDITIONS Food poisoning, Nausea, Poisoning, Travel sickness.

KEY SYMPTOMS Deathly nausea, with white pallor, cold perspiration on the face and a great sinking feeling in stomach. Great weakness and trembling. Feeling as if could die. Travel sickness.
COMPARE Arsenicum album, Cocculus, Nux vomica, Veratrum album.

URTICA URENS stinging-nettle

CONDITIONS Allergies, Breast issues, Burns, Hives.
KEY SYMPTOMS For simple burns, with only a little blistering. Pains are stinging, burning. For absence of milk in the breast, swelling of breasts. Allergic reactions on skin with hives, e.g. to shellfish and stinging, burning pains, at times with pains in the joints.
COMPARE Apis, Cantharis, Rhus tox.

VERATRUM ALBUM White Hellebore

CONDITIONS Cholera, Diarrhea, Food poisoning, Poisoning, Shock.
KEY SYMPTOMS The second remedy, after Arsenicum album for food/water poisoning, where there is great nausea, vomiting and diarrhea, often at same time. Feeling of coldness and cold perspiration on forehead with diarrhea.
COMPARE Arsenicum album, Nux vomica, Tabacum.

Topical remedies

The following remedies can be taken topically in either a tincture or creams/lotions.

ARNICA Excellent for bruising of parts and sore muscles and joints. It is however not to be used if the skin is broken.

CALENDULA The first remedy for any cuts, abrasions and lacerations. It is to be used in tincture to wash any wound and in cream to help the healing process. It acts as an antiseptic and healing agent. (It is often mixed with Hypericum (called Hypercal)).

EUPHRASIA This is used in tincture form for all sorts of eye problems, including conjunctivitis. Can be used with Hamamelis.

HAMAMELIS This is used to apply locally to piles and for injuries, similar to Arnica and in tincture in eye problems, including foreign objects in the eye.

RHUS TOX/RUTA These are both used for injuries and soreness to joints and muscles.

URTICA URENS This is used for hives on the skin and also for 1st degree burns. It can be mixed with Cantharis for more serious burns to the skin.

Herbal and Plant remedies and Essential Oils

Essential oils can be used either topically, neat or diluted; inhaled in steam or taken as a gargle. They may be taken in a compress form. Aromatherapists use essential oils for massage. They should not be taken internally. Certain oils need to be mixed in an oil base in the proportion of 20% or less as they may irritate the skin. The proportions can be much less, even as low as about 2% of the volume of base oil. These oils include eucalyptus, ginger, lemon, peppermint, pine and thyme. Lavender and tea tree oil can be given undiluted but any irritation should still be looked for. Citronella can be used directly, along with eucalyptus as an insect repellant. However, it shouldn't be used in children under the age of three and if there are any adverse reactions they should be stopped. Both citronella and eucalyptus need to be applied every 30-60 minutes for maximum effect against mosquitoes and other insects.

There are other oils which are not mentioned here and if used should be checked regarding the amounts to be used. Of the oils mentioned eucalyptus should be used in moderation due to its potential toxicity. Water-based gels can also be used to dilute essential oils. Compresses can be hot, and used for aches, pains and abscesses, or cold and used for headaches, bruises and acute sprains.

Avoid taking strong oils such as camphor and eucalyptus when taking homeopathy at the same time. The bottles should also be stored in a separate place from the homeopathic remedies.

Goldenseal should not be taken by pregnant and breast feeding women. It should not be taken for more than two weeks in one go. Those with high blood pressure or heart conditions should not use it and if on certain medications like SSRI antidepressants, it should be taken with caution and not for long periods.

Herbal medicines can be taken in tinctures or capsule form for convenience, but if possible taken in a fresh tea form which is often more effective and cheaper. This is for leaf-based herbal preparations. Harder, more woody herbs need to be decocted by breaking down and boiling until ready. Tinctures can be taken as directed on the bottle and are a good way to use herbal products when traveling.

Essential Oils

The following are a few of the most useful essential oils.

CITRONELLA OIL This has powerful insect repellant qualities and should be used along with eucalyptus to repel mosquitoes and other insects.

EUCALYPTUS OIL This has distinct antibacterial, antiviral, immune stimulant and also insect repellent qualities. It is used to help with colds, influenza, respiratory tract infections, and on the skin to prevent infections. It is a mouth wash but is not to be digested. It should be used on the skin, along with citronella as an insect repellant. It can be applied to inflamed muscles and joints. (A recent clinical trial using eucalyptus maculate citrodora – a combination of essential oils under the name Incognito has been proven to be effective in preventing bites of malarial mosquitoes and hence outbreaks of malaria). Whether a simple combination of eucalyptus and citronella is as effective is unknown but the proven ability of these oils to offer some resistance to mosquito bites is clear.

LAVENDER OIL Used as an antiseptic and anti-inflammatory, it can be used directly on the skin in burns, including sunburn, and scalds and bruises as well as for acne, eczema, dandruff and athletes foot. It can be used externally for muscle aches, pain and arthritic inflammations.

OREGANO OIL Used as an essential oil topically to heal cold sores and relieve rashes, bites, poison ivy and also applied to relieve muscle aching and can be a good insect repellant. (See below for more general use)

TEA TREE OIL Used against bacterial, viral and fungal infections. It can be used directly on the skin. Externally it is useful for fungal eruptions and for injuries due to its antimicrobial action. It is one of the most widely used essential oils.

Herbs and Plant remedies

Most of the following herbs are also used as homeopathic remedies. However they have specific herbal uses and so are listed separately here. Some are given their latin name and some their common name, depending mostly on how they are commonly called.

ARTEMESIA ANNUA sweet wormwood qingaosu. This has a distinct anti-parasitic action and is therefore used in the treatment of malaria and also babesia complications in Lyme disease. The extract Artemisinin is used as part of the combination therapy CAT for malaria. Evidence suggests though that the whole plant is effective both for malaria and other conditions, such as hemorrhoids, bilharzia, chronic dysentery.

It can also be used prophylactically against malaria (see **www.anamed.net** for information). It can be used both in a herbal form (a tea made by pouring one liter over approximately 2-5 grams (5 grams being the maximum dose) of dried leaves (10-25 grams of fresh leaves) and one cup taken 4 times a day), or in a homeopathic form, diluted to 6c potency in the treatment of babezia and malaria.

CRANBERRY It is used to help with bladder infections.

ECHINACEA purple cone – flower. This is used for the first stages of infection, whether viral or bacterial. It also helps to stimulate the immune system. It is good for blood poisoning.

ELDERBERRY sambucus nigra. It has effects on the respiratory system and also the kidneys. It has antiviral qualities and is effective in colds and influenza, especially when the respiratory system is involved and with much snuffling and cold symptoms. It contains high levels of Vitamin C.

EUCALYPTUS blue gum–tree. It has strong antiseptic qualities. It works on digestive disorders, catarrhal processes and influenza. It can be given in malaria and typhoid, any condition with relapsing fevers. It is useful in kidney conditions as a result of influenza.

GOLDENROD solidago virga. This is a very useful support for bladder and kidney infections, including kidney stones. It is also a good cleanser of the lymph.

GOLDENSEAL hydrastis. This is used for many conditions, including digestive problems, diarrhea, sinus and chest conditions, fungal infections of skin, eye irritation.

(It should not be taken by pregnant or breast feeding women or people with high blood pressure or heart conditions). It is taken internally for digestive conditions, including diarrhea. It can be used as a salve, tincture or powder.

MANGO mangifera indica. Mango leaves can be used in a tea form for diarrhea and ripe mangoes eaten in cases of amoebic dysentery.

MILK THISTLE OR LADY'S THISTLE silybum marianum. This is excellent to support the liver in many liver conditions, including hepatitis. It is also an antioxidant.

NEEM margosa bark - azadirachta indica. This has a distinct action as a prevention and also treatment of malaria. It is widely used as a food and medicine and has anti bacterial and anti viral action and is an important 'heal all' in many cultures, especially in Ayurvedic Medicine in India. It is put into toothpaste/powder and the twigs are used as brushes. It has distinct action on the skin, as an ointment or oil, being used for athlete's foot and other fungal infections, including candida and ringworm, scabies and for wounds and burns.

OREGANO OIL wild oregano - Origanum vulgare It has unique anti-bacterial, viral, fungal and parastic qualities. Used topically for fungal and viral skin conditions and internally for herpes, UTI's, amoebas (giardia), Shigella.

PAPAYA pawpaw - carica papaya. This has many health benefits, and the parts used are the skin, seeds and sap from an unripe papaya. Eating papayas in the tropics is excellent for digestive health as well as necessary vitamins. The sap is used to treat worms and indigestion and the leaves (as a tea) can be used for diarrhea and malaria. Unripe sap, mixed with clean water and salt can be used on wounds and for fungal infections. Also ripe papaya and/or the skin can be placed on wounds. (The sap can be obtained by making vertical cuts into an unripe papaya while it is still on the tree. Collect the sap into a cup (about 4 tsp for an adult and 1-2 tsp for a child). Ensure the knife is clean and wash the papaya first). Mix the sap into clean water, both for topical use and for taking internally.

ST. MARY'S THISTLE carduus marianus. This is a specific remedy for the liver and spleen. It assists in any inflammation, swelling and pain in the liver, whether due to acute hepatitis or chronic problems of the liver due to alcoholism and for spleen affections. Given in both tincture and homeopathic form.

TEASEL dipsacus. A common plant which is effective in the treatment of Lyme disease and other bacterial conditions.

UVA URSI bearberry. This is used in urinary conditions against bladder infections.

VALERIAN valeriana. This is good for general states of anxiety, nervousness, nerve pains and insomnia.

VERVAINE verbena officianalis. This helps lactating women produce more milk. It is also good for general exhaustion and nervousness, headaches and also upset digestion.

Index Of Conditions

Richard Pitt has practiced homeopathy for over 30 years. He has been involved with homeopathic education for many years, running a school in San Francisco for 12 years, and also teaching throughout the country as well as working for the development of standards of practice and education in the United States. He has written many articles for leading homeopathic journals, both in Europe and North America and is also Editor of an online journal, the California Homeopath (www.californiahomeopath.com). This manual has been extracted from a larger book, *The Natural Medicine Guide for Travel and Home* (www.thenaturalmedicineguide.com). He is the author of a homeopathic textbook, *Comparative Materia Medica, Integrating New and Old Remedies* and a book on the homeopathic study of tobacco.

He has spent over nine years traveling the world, much of this time in India and parts of Africa. He has been involved in three different projects in Africa, including establishing a school in Ghana and working in an integrative medical clinic, and helping to establish a homeopathic clinic in Malawi. In Kenya he has been working with an existing homeopathy school, helping in the educational development of students and graduates of the school and is now Educational Director of the school. He has been working with homeopaths throughout the world, including Brazil, India, U.K, Australasia and North America. He can be found at richardpitthomeopathy.com and at richardwpitt@gmail.com.